IT'S SIMPLE

MINERALS HEAL

LIDGEA CREERY MA

It's Simple

EAT DIRT

Make minerals part of your diet.

Creery, Lidgea
    It's Simple Minerals Heal
    ISBN- 13-978-1976463273
    ISBN-1976463270

Authors web page:
    https://sites.google.com/site/authorlidgeacreery/

Publisher: Amazon Create Space

Printed in the United States of America

Other Books by this Author

It's Simple:
    Vitamins Heal
    Minerals Heal
    Phenol Compounds (coming soon)

DEDICATION

To my Lord Jesus Christ,
My rock and my foundation,
Who brightens up the darkness.

Table of Contents

Minerals

Aluminum 15
Arsenic 20
Bismuth 21
Boron 23
Calcium 32
Chlorine 39
Chromium 45
Copper 47
Fluorine 51
Germanium 55
Gold 57
Iodine 58
Iron 61
Lithium 67
Magnesium 68
Manganese 68
Molybdenum 79
Phosphorus 81
Potassium 84
Selenium 88
Silicon 82
Silver 94
Sodium 100
Strontium 103
Sulfur 105
Vanadium 110
Zinc 113

Trace Minerals

Water 122
Electrolytes 127
Fulvic Acid Humic Acid 130
Shilajit 137
Smectite - Kaolinite Clay Groups 139

DISCLAIMER

The opinions expressed in this book are based upon my personal views and a reflection of my own ongoing investigation as connected to health, nutrition and disease. The information is not complete, nor does it cover all possible uses, benefits, diseases, actions, physical conditions, precautions, side effects, scientific research, nor other possible conditions or treatments.

The information contained in this book is general in nature and for discussion purposes only. The information is made available with the understanding that the author and publisher are not engaged in rendering medical, health, psychological or any other kind of personal or professional advice or services. It does not provide health or medical advice, nor should it be relied upon in part or in its entirety as the foundation for any medical decision.

This information is not to be used for self-diagnosis or self-treatment. It is not to be used as a substitute for qualified, professional medical advice. One should always consult their physician and other competent medical and health professionals regarding health, nutrition, diet, disease, ailment, physical conditions and medical treatment.

No warranties or guarantees are implied or expressed by the author or publisher. The author or publisher disclaim all responsibility for any liability, for any loss or risk, whether it be personal or otherwise, which is a direct or indirect consequence incurred by the use of any of the information from this book.

Our position and rights are consistent: You are accountable for your own beliefs, inferences, choices, actions and consequences.

INTRODUCTION

Does modern medicine have all the answers?

Haven't you ever wondered if modern drugs aren't really covering up the symptoms and not healing the real problem?

I believe that at times this may be the case. Then again, they do have quick fixes for many health problems. But are they really good for our bodies?

What's the alternative if we don't use these modern pharmaceutical cures?

Is there any other choice?

In some cases, I believe so, especially in prevention.

Is what is written in this book QUICK FIXES to medical problems?

No. I don't claim to have any quick fixes.

Foods containing minerals don't usually work rapidly. I encourage one to eat homegrown organic fruits and vegetables which might have more minerals than mass produced grocery store produce. By creating a healthier eating lifestyle, one might experience better health in time. By the way, juicing fruits and vegetables seems to get good results.

Some people want guarantees. This book doesn't have any. It shows you what research claims. With organically grown, mineral-rich foods and herbs, it's still a natural process in which what may help one person, yet might not work for another. All one can say is there seems to be a lot of research and truth out there that seems to show that there our food choices definitely affect our health and the possibility of having disease.

In this book, in "Possible Uses", some information is based in research and facts, as well as, alternative, traditional or folk lore remedies. When there are no scientific research found, you will note, no footnote numbers next to these items. But another twist is some scientific research will investigate folk lore remedies. Those, I have given footnotes. Where there are no footnotes listed, they might be used in alternative medicines, traditional medicines or as folk lore remedies. If pharmaceutical companies can't patient it and make money off of it, they aren't going to research it. Right?

Just like modern medicines, sometimes alternative remedies work, sometimes they don't, and sometimes they may work for one person but not for another and they too, may have some undesirable side effects, especially if used with incompatible drugs or nutrients.

But as for the author, I am willing to look at alternative uses for minerals, even folk lore remedies. Maybe the old-timers knew more about foods and herbs than modern people do. Maybe they've seen them work before and that's why the remedies have been passed down through generations. I remember my grandmother soaking her feet in Epsom Salt. She said it helped her feet to not hurt. Now, through my research, I found this folk lore remedy to have relevance.

I share this information with you, not stating that it is absolute truth but only that it might contain truth. I have tried to share with you, the reader, some of the warnings and hope that you will do your own research, and as always, it is at all times best to seek out the care of your physician to advise you.

How to Use this Resource!

In each segment of this book, I list several different areas of importance, which shall be discussed below.

Possible Uses

This section discloses some possible physical/emotional/ mental health concerns for which the mineral and related foods are used.

I do not claim anything to be a cure, that's up to the medical profession. But some of these "Possible Uses" health issues used can be scientifically proven as beneficial, some make sense based on their properties, and some are based on folk lore, traditional use, unverified but may be useful, or maybe some may not even work at all, that's why I list it as "Possible Uses". This may serve as a possible resource in guiding you as you do your own research.

In the "Possible Use" area, I often use research to verify the possible health benefits for the mineral. But sometimes the research isn't specific as to where the mineral came from; how the mineral was introduced into the body; whether it was tested on a human, animal, or a petri dish or what the result of the testing was. As you can see, there are a lot of variables. Please don't assume what the research is but seek out the truth for yourself, then consult with your physician. I do not profess having the answers. This is just a tool for you to explore the possibilities.

Possible Benefits

This contains what possible effects the mineral might have on the body. I found a variety of information among resources, so again, I list it as "Possible Benefits".

Properties

Properties are the attributes, character or qualities the mineral contains. This is not a conclusive list because of the lack of consistency in many other resources. My properties may vary from other resources, as often those resources may vary one from another.

Warnings, Precautions, and Side Effects

Most of the natural food sources shouldn't cause any problems unless one has an allergy or uses in excess. Often the problems come in when one is using supplements or using the food as a drug and not just a food. It is always best to check with one's medical professional before changing one's diet or overloading a food product in an effort to use it as a drug.

I have not found all the warnings for this section, so my hope is that you will be careful, prudent and use the mineral in moderation, and do your own research. When trying a new food, one should always pay attention to how the food may affect oneself. And when one tries a new food, it's wise to not overdo it, and if there is a problem, to definitely, see your doctor.

Food Sources

I did the best I can at finding food sources for each mineral. I realize there are a great many food items that have been left out, especially with herbs. I will be disclosing more about herbs later, in greater detail in another book coming up later.

The asterisk symbol "*" in the "Food Sources" section means "Best of the Rest", otherwise, more nutritious foods or ones with a higher mineral concentration.

Research

I have tried to find some research to show you how the mineral may affect you. I didn't usually research the simple things like allergies, digestion, headaches, skin problems, or stomach aches. But instead, I tried to focus on the more serious ailments like cancer, diabetes, heart disease, or radiation poisoning.

The information was gathered mostly from the scientific abstracts and not from the complete articles. Therefore, if one finds that information interesting or possibly relevant to you, you can order the complete article to see if it might be of value to you. I have given those references. Sometimes, I have found research that will contradict another individual's research. So again, sometimes facts don't always equate into truth.

It has been recommended that one uses research that is less than five years old. I have used older research, as well as newer research. If research is based upon truth, it doesn't vary. What is true today, was true in the past, and will remain true in the future. So, I tried to search for it, no matter what year it was done. If you come across some old research I have placed in here, it gives you the opportunity to check to see if some newer research is available which might shed more details and insight. And if you do find something that you believe might be valuable, remember to check with your medical professional.

MINERALS

So, what are these minerals?
Not surprisingly, the minerals we should be utilizing are found on the Periodic Table of Elements. And the truth is our body needs a lot of them, not in bulk, but mostly in trace, or very minute amounts.

Why?
99% of our body is made of minerals.

99% of Americans are deficient in organic trace minerals.

Our bodies need approximately 60 minerals to help us remain disease free.

Each mineral has certain jobs to do in our body…and if we don't have them, our bodies won't function properly.

What is the best way to get these necessary minerals?
Preferably, we should be getting minerals from the foods we eat. But because much of our soil is nutrient depleted, we may need to seek other sources, like supplements or trace mineral sources like healthier salt, mineral water, or clay, which will be discussed later.

Why Do We Need Minerals?

They are necessary to live. Without them we would die.

- Minerals are involved in transportation, activation, development, and maturation of immune cells, thus stabilizing the immune system, disease prevention, and so much more.

CATEGORIES OF MINERALS

Nonmetals

Halogens
- Highly reactive.
- All form acids when bonded to hydrogen, mineral salts.
- They are all toxic, harmful and lethal, external use only.
- Bromine, chlorine, fluorine, iodine, etc.

Nonmetals
- Don't conduct electricity or heat.
- Low melting point.
- Low density.
- Form acidic oxides.
- Dull and brittle in solid form.

Semimetals

Metalloids
- Difficult to classify, as they lie in between being metal and nonmetals.
- Have a metallic appearance.
- Brittle but are fair electrical conductors.
- Arsenic, boron, germanium, silicon, etc.

Metals

Alkali metals
- Exhibit well-characterized homologous actions.
- Soft, shiny, high reactive metals.
- Effortlessly cut with a knife.
- React to water.
- Lithium, potassium, sodium, etc.

Alkaline earth metals
- Soft, shiny, silvery white color.
- All alkaline earth metals are found in nature.
- Low density and melting point.
- React to water, forming strong alkaline hydroxides, except beryllium.
- Barium, beryllium, calcium, magnesium, strontium, radium.

Transition metals
- Paramagnetic
- Two or more oxidative states.
- Colored compounds.
- Heterogeneous and homogeneous catalytic activities.
- Conducts electricity.
- High density and melting point.
- Chromium, cobalt, copper, gold, iron, manganese, molybdenum, nickel, silver, vanadium, zinc, etc.

Post-transition metals
- Metallic elements.
- Poor metals.
- High boiling point and conductivity.
- Aluminum, bismuth, lead, tin, etc.

MINERALS & TRACE MINERALS

Aluminum   (Al)

- Post-transition metals element.

  Ann Louise Gittleman, a well-known nutritionist, calls aluminum a "detrimental protoplasmic poison."

- Some scientists feel it's not very toxic. Afterall, it's not a heavy metal because it doesn't act like lead or mercury.

Properties
- Conducts electricity and heat, corrosive-resistant, lightweight, strong

Possible Detriment
- ADD/ADHD, aging aortic tissue and arteries (less elastic), cancer, chronic constipation, colic, digestion, gastrointestinal problems, peptic ulcers, learning disorders[1], senile dementia[2], skin rashes.
- Alzheimer's disease[3], brain neurofibrillary tangle[4], impaired cognitive state[5], Parkinsonism-dementia[6]
- Aluminum starts in the stomach to be absorbed then deposited the brain's gray matter, increasing neurotransmitter breakdown, decreasing neurotransmitter reuptake, and slowing axonal transport.[7]
- High concentrations might be found in the brain, liver, lungs, and thyroid.
- Aluminum absorbed in the stomach, permeates the gut barrier and is deposited into the bone.[8]
- Aluminum leaches into acidic foods, like tomatoes or rhubarb.

- Fluoridated water used in aluminum cookware intensifies the aluminum in the water and food.
- Aluminum salts in deodorants can clog underarm lymph nodes, may cause breast problems, like breast cancer[9], might try natural baking soda, vinegar, oil or another natural deodorant instead.
- Antacids containing aluminum hydroxide, binds pepsin and weakens digestion of protein, also has astringent qualities, drying tissues and mucous linings, contributing to constipation.
- In some tap water, aluminum is used as an anti-clouding agent and chlorine kills good and bad bacteria.

Aluminum Compounds[10]
- Aluminum ammonium sulfate - cooking Alum
  - Food additive.
- Aluminum chloride
  - Antiperspirants
- Aluminum chlorohydrate
  - Antiperspirant
- Aluminum hydroxide
  - Antacid
  - Water purification.
- Aluminum sulfate
  - Food additive.
  - Water purification.

You could be eating it in your cookies and pickles or drinking it in your water.

Possibly Used as:
- Buffering agent, non-caking agent.

Aluminum & Aluminum Salts Sources
- added to some sea salt
- aluminum pans

- aluminum soda pop cans
- antacids
- aspirins, sleeping pills, buffered
- baking alum
- bread
- cocoa
- dental cement, false teeth bases
- food additives
- medical shots
- processed cheese
- some leafy vegetables
- tea
- white and refined flour
- aluminum foil
- antiperspirants
- baked goods
- baking powder
- children's sweets
- common table salt
- deodorants
- many cosmetics
- OTC medications
- some children's buffered aspirins
- some soy-based infant formulas
- vaccines

Warnings, Precautions, and Side Effects
Toxicity
- Corrosive agent on alimentary canal living tissue
- May bind to DNA
- Destroys vitamins in food
- Binds with other substances, like fluoride, calcium, or iron
- Do not put milk, vinegar, sauerkraut, potato salad, into an aluminum container.
- Aluminum may decrease the absorption of phosphorus and selenium in the gastrointestinal tract.
- Bone loss can lead to osteomalacia, a softening of the bone.
- Colitis attacks (putrid and zygotic) have been eliminated by changing cookware.
- Hepatic (liver) and nephritic (kidney) have also improved by changing cookware.
- Still debated as to how aluminum functions or interferes with the body.

• Has been correlated with weakened tissue of the gastrointestinal tract.

• In Alzheimer's disease, facts show there are higher aluminum levels in the brain tissue, called "neurofibrillary tangles," reducing nerve synapses and conduction.

Kitchenware test

• Boil non-chlorinated water in aluminum sauce pan or dish for 1/2 hour.

• Pour water into a clear bowl.

• You will see aluminum remnant in water.

• 4-5 grains of aluminum is ingest with each meal.

Possible Symptoms of Toxicity

- anorexia
- diarrhea
- dry mucous membranes
- head colds
- heartburn and nausea
- joint pain
- low energy
- paralytic muscular conditions
- throbbing headache
- weakness
- brain functioning
- dry skin
- gastrointestinal inflammation, colic
- head pain with constipation
- heaviness
- kidney and liver problems
- muscle twitching
- profound numbness
- vertigo

Children's Toxicity Effects of High Aluminum

• Brain disease in children with kidney disease.

• Bone disease in children with kidney disease.

Possible Treatment for Toxicity

Check with doctor.
- Decrease contact with it.
- Oral chelating, Tetracycline is a mild aluminum chelator.
- Calcium disodium edetate (EDTA) is fairly nontoxic and binds to clear aluminum.
- Deferoxamine, an iron chelator, also binds to aluminum.
    - A study shows a 40% improvement with Deferoxamine.
- Deferoxamine, malic acid, citric, and succinic acids excreted aluminum.[11]

Experiment to detect Aluminum
- Take an aluminum bowl or a bowl with aluminum foil inside.
- Add 1 c. water.
- Next add 3 T. sodium bicarbonate (baking soda).
- When the baking soda (alkaline) is added, it melts becoming a gas.
- It's presumed this causes poisoning, possibly causing gastro-intestinal problems, renal or hepatic degeneration.

Arsenic   (As)

- Non- metal, Metalloid.
- Metallic form is brittle and tarnishes. The nonmetallic form is less reactive.
- Not essential.
- Found in the earth in small concentrations.
- Can be found in groundwater, in conjunction with sulfur.

Possible Uses
- Glass making, herbicides, insecticides, insomnia, itchy skin, pesticides, promyelocytic leukemia[12], psoriasis, sickle cell disease[13], skin cancer, wood preservation

Warning, Precautions and Side Effects
- Deadly poison.
- 10 mcg/kg/day over time of organic arsenic can cause arsenic poisoning.[14]
- Organic arsenic has been shown to reduce children's intelligence test scores.
- Lung, skin, stomach and intestinal irritation.
- Can reduce the resistance to infections.
- Decrease red and white blood cells.
- Can cause infertility and miscarriage.
- Can damage DNA. [15]
- Arsenic trioxide treatment can cause skin rash and hyperglycemia.[16]
- Might cause chronic hepatitis, cirrhosis, noncirrhotic portal hypertension and liver hemangiosarcoma.[17]
- Can cause basal cell carcinoma, bladder cancer, Bowen's disease, brain damage, heart problems, hyperkeratosis, keratosis, lung cancer and skin cancer and squamous-cell carcinoma squamous-cell carcinoma.

Bismuth   (Bi)

- Post-transition metal.
- Heavy metal like arsenic and lead, but not as toxic.
- Not essential.
- Bismuth and lithium are often paired together.

Possible Uses
- AIDS/HIV diarrhea[18], bloody/mucous stools, campylobacter pyloridis[19], cosmetics, diarrhea, eye infections, gastric ulcers, gastrointestinal disorders, heartburn, helicobacter pylori[20], medicines, peptic ulcers[21], Pseudomonas aeruginosa[22], respiratory tract infection[23], SARS coronavirus[24], staphylococci[25], stomachache, traveler's diarrhea

Possible Benefits
- Reduces acidity.
- Absorbs toxins.

Properties
- Anti-diarrhea, anti-ulcer, antibacterial, antimicrobial

Warning, Precautions and Side Effects
- Do not take if pregnant or breast feeding, check with physician.
- Avoid if you have allergies to bismuth.
- Do not take if you have a rash or itching.
- Do not take if you have bleeding or breathing problems.
- Can cause kidneys damage, liver damage.
- Can cause colitis, encephalopathy, headache, hearing problems, hypoadrenalism, mental confusion, muscle twitching, slurred speech, staggering gait, tremors, visual problems.

- Overdose can cause dark tongue, gums, stool, and a metallic taste.
- Subsalicylates can cause bleeding, if using with ulcers, check with physician.

Overdose
- Use calcium.
- See physician.

Food Sources
- Mineral water, roots, tubers, sea vegetables

Other Sources
- Bismatrol, Bismuth Subsalicylate, Diotame, Kao-tin, Kaopectate®, Maalox®, Peptic Relief, Pepto Relief, Pepto-Bismol®, Pink Bismuth, Total Relief®

Boron   (B)
Organic boron   Sodium borate
Cheated boron   Boric Acid

- Metalloid element.

Possible Benefits
- Helps make vitamin D active.
- Might increase calcium absorption.
- Reduces calcium excretion from the body.
- Builds bones and increases bone mineral density.
- Strong enzyme inhibitor for cancer.
- Lowers plasma lipid levels.
- Activates estrogen.
- Helps concentration, eye-hand coordination and short-term memory.
- Affects steroid hormonal levels.
- Delivery agent for cancer treatment.[26]
- Affects characteristics of cell membrane and the signaling transmembrane.[27]
- Affects hormone processes at the cellular membrane level.[28]
- Its half-life is 1 day so it doesn't stay in the tissue long but does stay in the bone.[29]

Boron Food Sources
- Almonds, apples, avocados, banana, beans, borlotii beans, broccoli, chickpeas, currants, dates, dried beans, fruits, hazel nuts, honey, kiwi, leafy green vegetables, lentils, nuts, olive, onion, oranges, peanuts, pears, pecans, potatoes, plum, prunes, pulses, raisins, red apples, red grapes, red kidney beans, soybeans, sultana, tomato, vegetables, whole grains

• The amount of boron in the foods is dependent upon how much boron is in the ground while the plant is being grown.

Research

U.S. Department of Agriculture study reported that when postmenopausal women take 3 milligrams of boron per day, they lose 1/3rd less magnesium, 40% less calcium and a little bit less phosphorus through their urine.[30]

Evidence is mounting in showing the bioactive benefits of boron. Reports express that this mineral might be an essential mineral, for its actions help with arthritis, bone growth, bone maintenance, the central nervous system functioning, the reduction of cancer risk, facilitates the hormones, improves the immune response, reduces inflammation and modulates oxidative stress. Some data suggests that human should limit intake to less than 1.0 mg/day.[31]

Boric acid

• Contains boron, oxygen, and hydrogen (H_3BO_3).
• In nature, boron doesn't exist alone but is combined with other common elements.
• Occurs naturally in water and soil.

What is Boric acid?
• Made by uniting borax and sulfuric acid.
• Boron compound of mineral and salt, boric acid.
• Boric acid crystals are white, odorless, and nearly tasteless, looks like fine table salt.

- Used as a buffer in pharmaceutical preparations.
- Boric acid and other borates are used as a source of boron in over-the-counter nutritional supplements.
- Boric acid should not be ingested in its natural form but only used as a manufactured supplement.

Borax
Sodium borate   Sodium tetraborate
Disodium tetraborate

Historical Perspective

- Speculated that China used it around 900 A.D. to enhance ceramic container glazing properties.
- Arabians preserved gold and silver finish during fabrication.
- In 1702, Wilhelm Homberg created man-made boric acid crystals.
- In 1870's, borax deposits were discovered in Nevada and Death Valley, California.
- In 1949, Silly Putty® was created by mixing silicone oil with boric acid.
- Used for a centuries to cleanse and treat burns, scrapes, skin irritations, wounds of all kinds.

Possible Uses of Boron/Boric Acid
- Allergies, aluminum chloride-induced neurotoxicity[32], anti-aging preparations, arthritis[33], aspergilliosis[34], attention[35], azole-refractory C GLABRATA vaginitis[36], bacterial vaginosis[37], body building, bone health[38], bone strength, brain function[39], breast cancer[40], cancer, candida albicans[41], candida vaginitis[42], canker sores, cholesterol control, cervical cancer[43], cleaning agent, chronic mycotic

vaginal infections[44], coccidiodomycosis[45], cognitive performance[46], colon cancer, congestive heart failure[47], contact lens solution, coronary heart disease, cosmetics, Cryptococci meningitis[48], curing agent, detergent, diabetes (topical)[49], diabetic neuropathy (topical)[50], diabetic ulcers[51], Ehrlich ascites carcinoma[52], enamel glazes, eye disinfectant, eye-hand coordination[53], female problems, fire retardant, food preservative, forge welding flux, flame retardant, fluoride chelator, fungal meningitis[54], foot-and-mouth disease, gold extraction, herpes virus[55], histoplasmosis[56], hoof rot, hoof thrush[57], hyperthyroidism, insect control, joint health[58], lung cancer (women smokers)[59], manual dexterity[60], menopause, metallurgy, mice deterrent, mineral retention, non-diabetic ulcers, neutron-capture shield for radiation, onychomycosis[61], oral candida/thrush[62], osteoarthritis[63], osteoporosis[64], pH buffering agent, pink eye, prostate cancer[65], radiation neutron absorber (elemental boron), reproduction, rheumatoid arthritis[66], short /long-term memory[67], skin inflammation, tinea corpora[68], tinea pedis[69], tinea versicolor[70], tooth bleaching, torulopsis glabrata vaginitis[71],vaginitis bacterial infection[72], vulvovaginal candidiasis[73], woman's peri-menopausal hormones[74], wood preservative, wound infections, yeast infections

Possible Benefits of Boron/Boric acid
- Bioactive, speeds healing, prevents infection.
- Hormone facilitation.
- Immune response and inflammation reduction.
- Boron compounds slow down fungus growth and is dependable.
- Natural safe popular insect control, doesn't kill bugs but dehydrates a lot of insects by initiating tiny cracks in their exoskeletons, then they dry out.

- Kills ants, cockroaches, silverfish, termites, and other familiar household insects.
- Fairly non-toxic to people and pets unless used in toxic amounts, read the warning on label.
- Fortifies items against fire.
- Inhibits combustible gas release from burning in cotton, paper, and wood products and other cellulosic materials.
- Releases chemically bound water to reduce combustion.
- Boric acid and similar borates strengthen the temperature and chemical resistance of specialty glass like microwavable glassware, halogen light bulbs, plasma screens, skis, circuit boards, and fiberglass textiles.
- Hardens and treats steel alloys and aids in applying metal plating.

Boric Acid and Yeast Infections

- Sufficiently mild to wash the eye in small amounts.
- Candida and yeast over-growth infections are eliminated by boric acid.
- Boric acid aids in bringing back the vagina's alkaline ph-factor.
- Calms itching and burning, alleviates skin/vagina inflammation, and cleans the infected area to speed up healing.
- Some physicians recommend boric acid with a standard anti-fungal drug to alleviate a yeast infection, please council with your health practitioner.
- Vagisil is often used for a vaginal yeast infection, the main active ingredients is boric acid.

Possible Deficiency

- Abnormal bone growth.
- Increased urinary calcium excretion.

Properties

- Anti-infection, antibacterial[75], antibiotic, anticancer[76], antifungal[77], antineoplastic, antiprotozoal[78], antifungal[79], antimicrobial, antiviral[80], boromycin antibiotic, chemo preventive[81], chemotherapeutic[82], fungicidal, insecticide, proteasome inhibitor[83], very mild antiseptic

Warnings, Precautions, and Side Effects of Boron/Boric Acid

- Use in moderation.
- Foods with natural occurring boron will not cause an overdose.
- If the boric acid label says "inert ingredients", don't use it orally.
- Some baby powders may contain boric acid and might pose a risk to the infant.
- Some claim that boric acid is poison and should not be taken orally.

Mild overdose symptoms

- Approximately 15-20 mg daily.
- Diarrhea, epigastria pain, hematemesis, nausea, vomiting

Overdose symptoms

- Approximately 25 mg daily.
- Alopecia (hair loss), anorexia, convulsions, depression, dermatitis, desquamation, exfoliation, headaches, hyper excitability, inskin erythema, indigestion, irritability, lethargy, loose motions, nausea, vomiting, weakness and possibly skeletal abnormalities
- Do not use with kidney problems, can accumulate in brain, heart, kidneys and tissues.
- Do not overuse, 6 oz. can kill an adult, poisonous.
- Kills ants, cockroaches, and other insects by sprinkling powder where they go.

• Some pharmacies may have the pharmaceutical form of this chemical, often behind the counter but doesn't need a prescription.
• Boric acid poisoning is blue-green vomit, diarrhea, and bright red rash on skin.
• Other poisoning symptoms are blisters, collapse, coma, convulsions, drowsiness, fever, lethargy, low blood pressure, decreased urine output, sloughing of skin, twitching facial muscles, hands, legs and feet.[84]

Research

Stephen J Baker in his article, "Therapeutic potential of boron-containing compounds", believes that because there is lack of information about boron products in therapeutics. He believes over the next 10 years, there will be a great future for it in drug discovery.[85]

In this research, conventional antifungal agents were found to be ineffective against chronic mycotic vaginal infections. Boric acid was found to be successful in curing patients by 98%, even those who had used the conventional antifungal agents previously.[86]

Diabetic women with candida glabrata vulvovaginal when given vaginal suppositories with boric acid for 14 days, demonstrated a greater incidence of mycological fungal cure with boric acid than 150 mg of oral fluconazole.[87]

Patients preferred taking 600 mg of boric acid powder in a gelatin capsule for 7-10 days with a 92% cure rate, and a half-life of 12 hours, at the cost of 31 cents for fourteen capsules. The nystatin vaginal cream cure rate was 64% for the same amount of time. [88]

Boric Acid Folk Recipes

Laundry Soap
- 1/2 c. borax
- 1/2 c. washing soda
- 1/4 bar of graded ivory, Zote or Fels Naptha soap
- Optional:
    1/4 c. dry fabric softener
    1/4 c. dry oxygen (oxy…) fabric cleaner

Pink Eye Boric Acid Folk Remedy Wash
- 1/4-1 t. boric acid powder (should feel like water on eye, if it burns, cut down the boric acid)
- 2 c. hot water, let cool
- Wash eye out with cotton ball

Vaginal Yeast Infection Folk Remedy
- 1/8 c. of boric acid put into small 00 dissolvable gelatin capsules that are safe for vaginal insertion
- Insert 1 capsule daily for 7-14 days and infection should be gone
- If you find that the boric acid burns, it is best to err on the side of safety and reduce the amount of boric acid or seek other treatment.

Wound, Cuts, Abrasions
- Sprinkle a little boric acid powder on the cut and it should scab up quickly

Canker Sore Treatment
- Same as pink eye treatment
- Dip cotton ball in solution and place it on the sore

Boric Acid Adult Drink Folk Remedy
- 1/8 t. boric acid
- In 1 liter water
- Has been used to cure many things like candida yeast infection, arthritis, etc.
- Some people claim it works.

Herpes Virus Topical Folk Remedy
- Boric acid
- Aspirin
- Make paste with water or alcohol solution

Anti-fungal Topical Soap Folk Remedy
- New bar of glycerin soap melted
- 1/4 c. borax
- 10 drops tea tree oil
- Add together, put in form and let cool

Homemade Toothpaste
- 4 parts baking soda
- 2 parts Xylitol powder
- 4 parts coconut or olive oil
- Essential oil for flavor: cinnamon, citrus, mint, root beer, spearmint, wintergreen

Optional: For candida yeast infection or thrush, use a little boric acid in the solution.

Calcium   (Ca)

- Alkaline earth metal element.
- Must be taken daily, every cell in our body needs it, and our bones store it and release it when our blood has low calcium.
- Needs vitamin D to aid in its absorption, so get out into the sun.
- Vitamins C, E, K and the minerals magnesium, potassium and boron help the calcium absorption into the bones.
- Amino acid lysine is also needed for calcium absorption, particularly in the intestines.[89]
- Calcium and magnesium ratio is 2:1. They need to be taken together in the correct ratio to be beneficial.

Possible Uses

- ADD/ADHD[90], age-related bone loss, aluminum chelator, Alzheimer's[91], Alzheimer-type senile dementia[92], anxiety[93], bacillary meningitis[94], blood pressure control, bone/teeth strength, brain health, breast cancer[95], breathing trouble, cardiac arrhythmias[96], cardiopulmonary disease hypoxia dementia[97], cerebral helminthiasis[98], cerebrovascular dementia[99], childhood "growing" pain, cholesterol control, circulation, colon cancer[100], Cushing Syndrome hypoglycemia[101], depression[102], endocrine disease dementia[103], frequent bone fractures, heart palpitations, heart disease, heavy metal chelator, helps blood clotting, hip fracture prevention[104], hormone secretion, Huntington[105], hypertension (African descent & sodium use), hyperlipidemia[106], hyperthyroidism[107], hypothyroidism[108], hyperparathyroidism[109], hyperparathyroidism[110], hypocalcaemia[111], hypocalcaemia[112], hypoglycemia[113], hypopituitarism[114], infectious disease dementia[115], insomnia, lead chelator, leg cramps, liver disease[116], mood[117], mineral chelator, muscle

cramps, nervousness, numbness in arms/legs,
osteomalacia, osteoporosis[118], Pick disease[119], postmenopausal bone loss[120], prevents water retention,
Parkinson[121], regulates heartbeat, relaxes heart and
muscles, rheumatism, rickets, sinusitis, stunted teeth/bone
growth, syphilis helminthiasis[122], tooth decay, tubercular
meningitis[123], Wilson's[124]

Possible Benefit

- Needed for normal blood clotting.
- Extremely important because it circulates in soft body
tissue and blood, and if it becomes low, it steals calcium
from the bones, teeth, and nails, insufficient may lead to
death.
- Increases bone mineral density in children, adolescents,
women, men and the elderly.
- With correct calcium magnesium ratio, it helps reduce
blood cholesterol levels.
- Activates and stimulates things like:
  - DNA
  - Insulin
  - Nerve impulse transmissions
  - Potassium channels
  - Skeletal transport of glucose
  - Muscle contraction and relaxation
  - Enzymes
  - Proteins
  - Platelet mobility

Possible Deficiency

- Hypocalcemia tetany is low calcium.
- Hypocalcemia, low calcium, is nerves and muscle cells
become hyperactive. Symptoms may be involuntary
muscle spasms, muscle cramping, numbness, paresthesia
(burning, prickling sensations), Petechiae (tiny red dot
bleeding under skin), poor appetite, or Purpura (large
bruising).

- Hypercalcemia is when the calcium level is too high; therefore it depresses the immune system causing calcium deposits in blood vessels and kidneys.
- Symptoms may be back pain, bone pain, curved spine, height loss, neck pain

Possible Deficiency Life-Threatening Conditions[125]
- Fainting, loss of consciousness, not alert.
- Chest pain, heart palpitations, pressure.
- Irregular, rapid or weak pulse.
- Breathing problems, shortness of breath, wheezing, choking, not breathing, difficulty breathing.
- Seizures.
- Muscle contractions.
- Uncommon extreme weakness.

Warnings, Precautions, and Side Effects
- Pregnant women need more calcium.
- Do not take calcium with iron, it blocks it, so it is an iron chelator, which may be useful under certain conditions.
- Spinach has calcium but also has oxalic acid (reducing agent/chelator, 30 times stronger than acetic acid) which prevents calcium from being absorbed.
- Dried beans and peas also have phytic acid which combines with calcium and prevents it from being absorbed.
- Eating a lot of high-protein foods, meats, causes calcium to decrease more by exiting through the urine.
- Strict vegetarians require 1/3 less calcium than meat eaters.
- Nightshade plants reduce calcium.
- Smoking can cause bone loss.
- Avoid high phosphorous, simple sugar, and animal protein, they deplete calcium in bones.

- Almonds, beet greens, cashews, chard, cocoa, kale, rhubarb, soybeans and spinach have oxalic acid and can interfere with calcium in the intestines.
- Calcium supplements shouldn't be used by people with kidney stones or kidney disease.
- Too much calcium can interfere with zinc absorption.
- Too little vitamin D, or too much phosphorus and magnesium hinders calcium uptake.
- Check your calcium supplement by putting it into a glass of water, if it doesn't dissolve within 20 minutes, you may want to change your brand.
- Calcium and magnesium can assist in getting rid of aluminum, don't use magnesium oxide or calcium carbonate, use an organic chelation like amino-acid chelation or citrate.

Possible Treatment
- Remember to use calcium with vitamin D.
- Eat food with calcium supplements.
- Bone meal, *calcium carbonate, dolomite, oyster shell.
- Take vitamin C with minerals, it increases its absorption.
- *Calcium carbonate is the one which is best absorbed.
- Numerous sites state that a bone which has sufficient calcium will block strontium 90 radioactivity since strontium 90 is chemically similar to calcium but didn't find evidence to verify that as fact.

Non-Dairy Food Sources
- Alfalfa, almonds, anise, asparagus, Atlantic Ocean perch, beans, beet greens, blackstrap molasses, blue crab, bone meal, brewer's yeast, bok choy, bone meal, broccoli, cabbage, calcium-fortified orange juice, canned salmon (eaten with bones), canned sardines (eaten with bones), carob, chard, clams, collards, dandelion greens, dark leafy greens, dolomite, dulse, farmed Rainbow trout, figs, firm tofu prepared with nigari, fortified ready-to-eat cereals, kale, kelp, leafy green vegetables, mustard greens, navy beans, nettle, oats, okra, Pak-choi, parsley, prunes, sardines, sea food, sesame seeds, soy beans, tofu, turnip greens, watercress, white beans
- Hard water

Dairy Food Sources
- Buttermilk, blue cheese, cheddar cheese, Colby cheese, feta cheese, goat's milk, milk, Monterey Jack cheese, mozzarella cheese, muenster cheese pasteurized process Swiss cheese, plain yogurt, provolone cheese, ricotta cheese, Romano cheese, Swiss cheese, whey

Research

In general, this study suggests that the role of calcium signaling is involved in cell membrane through a low-frequency electromagnetic field to aid the immune system of living organisms.[126]

Calcium elaborate solution placed in nose got rid of parainfluenza-3 virus within minutes.[127]

Calcium and Vitamin D is Key[128]

Carl J. Reich. M.D., back in the 1950s, asserted that civilizations diseases were caused by a chronic deficiency of calcium and vitamin D. He noticed his patients exhibiting over-stimulated autonomic nervous system symptoms: such as, acidic saliva, allergic nasal congestion (chronic), anxiety, bloating, coated tongues, chronic fatigue, constipation or diarrhea (chronic), easily broken finger nails, headaches, indigestion, muscle aches and cramping, night sweats, physical weakness, pins/needles sensations, psychosomatic (hypochondriac), restless legs, sleep problems, and spastic muscles.

He noticed their diets were high in acidic foods like meat and starches, high in sulfur and phosphorus, and low in vitamin D, such as, egg yolk, fish, liver, or sunlight. He also noticed they were low in alkaline foods like fruits, vegetables, foods high in calcium, magnesium, and potassium.

Dr. Reich stated that vitamin D effects calcium, making it "biologically active," therefore, making it available to the cell through 1000 plus enzymatic processes.

He further stated that when one is calcium deficient, it would starve the cell of energy, thus creating undesirable symptoms like allergies, anxiety, constipation, cracked nails, depression, diarrhea, fatigue, irritability, leg cramps, and muscle tenderness.[129]

Calcium Carbonate

Possible Uses
- Baking soda substitute, breast cancer[130], chronic renal failure undergoing dialysis[131], leavening agent, postmenopausal bone loss[132]

Possible Uses
- Lowers serum phosphorus.[133]
- Raises serum calcium.[134]

Recipe

Homemade Toothpaste
- 4 parts calcium carbonate or calcium magnesium powder
- 2 parts baking soda
- 2 parts Xylitol powder
- 4 parts coconut, olive, or sesame oil
- Essential oil for flavor: cinnamon, citrus, mint, root beer, spearmint, wintergreen

Chlorine   (Cl)

- A natural occurring gas.
- 3rd highest negatively-charged electrical element.

Possible Uses

- Bleach, disinfectant, gold ore extraction, kills waterborne infectious disease, plastic production, swimming pool sanitizer

Properties

- Anti-bacterial, disinfectant, fungicide, pesticide

What it does

- Kills cholera, some E. coli, typhoid germs.
- Kills bacteria, fungi, molds.
- Kills vitamin E, other vitamins, intestinal flora.
- Attacks DNA.
- Chlorine gas (bertholite) was a WWI weapon, sinks to lower levels, had a pineapple/pepper smell, attacked mucous lining in lungs, became hydrochloric acid, and was lethal.
- Iraq War, trucks with chlorine gas were detonated.

Warning, Precautions and Side Effects

- Do not mix with any other household product.
- Do not inhale.
- Has carcinogenic effects or mutagenic effects[135].
- May cause birth defects[136] and blindness.

What damage it can do.

- Bladder, colon, and liver damage/cancer.
- Chlorine gas-induced lung injury.
- Attacks eyes, mucous membrane and skin irritant.

- Can cause heart disease, hives, malformations in children.

How to neutralize Chlorine.
1. Leave chlorinated water out in the sun light for a day.
2. Carbon-based filtration system
3. Dechlorination tablets (vitamin C)
    - One 1000 mg. vitamin C or ascorbic acid will remove the chlorine from water in a bathtub or there is the Sonaki Vitamin C shower head, or there are chlorine filters that might remove the chlorine but not the chloramine.
    - Add orange peel slice and let sit for 30 minutes.
4. Boiling tap water eliminates chlorine. Short boil removes 30%.
5. Sodium thiosulfate
    - Declorinates chlorine from tap water.
    - Antidote to cyanide poisoning, antifungal for ringworm.
    - Management of chemotherapy extravasions.
6. Chloramine can be added to baths to instantly neutralize chlorine in water while providing sulfur for the vital sulfur pathways[137].

Remedy
For chlorine gas-induced lung injury.
- To improve lung function, use aerosolized terbutaline followed by aerosolized budesonide[138].

Research
Chlorinated drinking water has been associated with cancer. The chemicals in chlorination show carcinogenic potential.[139]

Few studies have been conducted on chlorinated solvents. TCE-contaminated drinking water might cause cardiac defects, choanal atresia, oral clefts and other possible birth defects but more studies are needed for follow-up.[140]

Chloramine (chlorine + ammonia)

Chloramine Benefits
- Disinfectant reduces pathogenic diseases.
- Hides the chlorine odor.

Warning, Precautions and Side Effects
- Irritates eyes, lungs, nose, skin and throat.
- Might contribute to asthma.
- Attracts lead from older plumbing.

How to neutralize the Chloramine's Ammonia.
1. Same as chlorine above.
2. Vinegar + ammonia = ammonium acetate.
   - Used as a food preservative, fungicide, insecticide, inhibits pathogens.
   - Do not inhale, may irritate nose, throat and lungs.
   - May burn eyes and skin.
3. Sodium by cation resin water softener or cation exchange resin in the hydrogen form.
4. Reverse Osmosis filter
5. Activated Carbon Water Filter
6. Ultraviolet light

Research
Chloramines, a chlorine and ammonia compound, commonly used urban water bactericidal agent and has been connected in two recent epidemics. It creates hemoglobin denaturation, inhibiting red cell metabolism reduction.[141]

Chloride

- Essential natural-occurring mineral.
- Water-soluble.
- An ion of chlorine.
- Essential electrolyte mineral, balances pH acid/alkaline imbalances.
- Chloride has 1 electron less than chlorine, which helps it bind to another element.
- Found in salts, like aluminum chloride, chloride bicarbonate, calcium chloride, lithium chloride, magnesium chloride, potassium chloride, sodium chloride, trospium chloride, zinc chloride, among others.

Possible Benefits
- Located in body fluids.
- Maintains acid/base balance.
- Transmits nerve impulses.
- Regulates fluids.
- The highest amount of chloride is found in red blood cells.
- Aids blood volume and pressure.
- Hydrochloric acid helps break down food in the stomach for digestion.
- Kidneys regulate chloride in the blood.
- Crosses the blood brain barrier.[142]

Magnesium Chloride "The Master Magnesium Compound"
- Unquestionable dietary and topical therapeutic uses, due to high effectiveness, fast acting, constant stability and effective action.
- Greater absorption bioavailability for magnesium because of the chloride.

- Chloride aids in hydrochloric acid production in stomach for better digestion, especially with declining gastric acid secretions, particularly for the elderly.
- Aids in the reduction of negative bacteria, viruses and yeast in the gastrointestinal area.
- Chloride aids in the absorption and assimilation of magnesium.
- Topical oil/spray or solution of magnesium chloride aids in wound cleansing and healing.
- Taken orally, it boosts the immune system.

Possible Chloride Deficiency
Hypochloremia
- Is when blood levels drop.

Symptoms
- Excessive fluid loss
  - Diarrhea
  - Heavy sweating
  - Vomiting
  - Overuse of coffee
  - Overuse of diuretics or laxatives
- Congestive Heart failure
- Addison's disease
- Some kidney disorders
- Can lead to alkalosis.
  - High blood pH.
  - Excessive potassium loss in urine.
  - Muscle control loss.
  - Breathing and swallowing difficulties.

Chloride Overdose
Hypernatremia
- High blood sodium levels.

Symptoms
- Excessive blood volume caused by excessive salt intake.
- Abdominal cramps
- Breathing problems
- Cardiovascular disease
- Convulsions
- Diarrhea
- Dizziness
- Fast/irregular heartbeat
- Feet/hands swelling
- Heightened blood pressure
- Increased heart rate
- Kidney disease
- Low blood pressure
- Nausea
- Reduced urine production
- Seizures
- Swelling (edema)
- Vomiting
- Coma
- Death

Warning, Precaution and Side Effects
- Artificial chloride isn't utilized by the body.
- Do not use potassium chloride with kidney failure, severe burns, tissue injury or Addison's disease.

Chloride Food Sources
- Bacon, celery, cheese, ham, kelp, lettuce, olives, preserved meats, rye, salt substitutes, sausages, sea salt, seaweed, some vegetables, table salt, tomatoes, yeast

Chromium   (Cr)
Chromium citrate   Chromium pictolinate
Chromium iodinate   High-chromium yeast

* Transitional metal element.
* Chromium pictolinate seems to be the easiest for the body to absorb.

Possible Uses
* Acne, Alzheimer's[143], aspergillus fumigatus[144], aspergillus niger[145], atherosclerosis[146], blood pressure control, blood sugar control[147], body fat, depression[148], candida albicans[149], coronary heart disease[150], diabetes (type 1, 2)[151], glaucoma, growth problems, heart problems, hypercholesterolemia[152], hyperglycemia[153], hypertension[154], hypoglycemia, malnourished[155], obesity[156], psoriasis, stroke, triglyceride control
* Gram-negative/positive bacteria might have high sensitivity to chromium, along with moderate antifungal activity.[157]

Possible Benefits
* Reduces food cravings, metabolizes carbohydrates, protein and fat.
* Conflicting results as to whether it may decrease body fat and foster lean muscles.
* Chromium picolinate seems to show promise at reducing body fat.
* Helps insulin to bind with cells and activates insulin receptors.[158]

Possible Deficiency
* Experts believe there is a chromium deficiency world-wide.
* Glucose intolerance intensifies with age.

- Refined sugar and processed foods contribute to chromium predicament.
- Gestational diabetes which briefly happens with pregnant women.

Properties
- Antibacterial, antifungal[159], antimicrobial, low cycotoxic

Warnings, Precautions, and Side Effects
- Can be very toxic, use according to supplement instructions.
- Can interfere or help with insulin so use with discretion.
- Refining wheat destroys chromium in wheat germ.
- Sugar depletes chromium.

Toxicity Symptoms
- Gastrointestinal ulcers, kidney damage, liver damage, rashes

Food Sources
- Brewer's yeast and wheat germ are rich in it.
- Black pepper, bran cereal, broccoli, brown rice, calves' liver, cheese, chicken, corn, corn oil, dairy products, dried beans, eggs, meats, molasses, mushrooms, onions, oysters, potatoes, thyme, tomatoes, whole grains, whole wheat
- Supplements are chromium citrate, chromium nictitate, chromium iodinate, high-chromium yeast but use in smaller quantities.

Research

Moderately dieting and exercising from African-American women lost a considerable amount of fat, without harming muscle by taking niacin-bound chromium. There seems to be no bad side effects from the 3 times daily intake of 200 µg of niacin-bound chromium over a 2 month period.[160]

Copper (Cu)

- Transitional metal element.
- Essential for good health.

Possible Uses

- Acute diarrhea[161], Alzheimer's[162], amyotrophic lateral Sclerosis (ALS - Lou Gehrig's disease) aortic aneurysms[163], brain development[164], avian influenza (H9N2)[165], blood vessel, bone strength[166], breast cancer[167], candida albicans[168], cardiovascular disease[169], cholesterol control, immune system, infection, irregular heartbeat, immune system[170], malnourished[171], myocardial contractility[172], nerves, neurodegenerative disease[173], osteoporosis[174], Parkinson's, Prion disease[175], prostate cancer[176], rheumatoid arthritis[177], wound healing[178]

Possible Benefits

- Drug transporter.
- Vital for hematologic, neurologic, skeletal and vascular systems.[179]
- Works with zinc and vitamin C to form elastin, and the healing process.
- More than a trace can be toxic but it seems our body naturally knows how to regulate it, because of this, deficiency and poisoning is uncommon.
- Part of a cell enzyme that is required for the release of energy.
- Needed for production of melanin, the dark pigment in hair and skin.
- Involved in iron metabolism, where iron can't be properly incorporated into blood.
- Vital factor in T-cells in the immune system.
- Helps body absorb and utilize iron.

- Part of a group of enzymes that help form hemoglobin and collagen.
- Component that neutralizes free radicals, called super oxide.
- Copper bracelets do have therapeutic value for arthritis inflammation.[180]
- Supports collagen's bone connective tissue.
- Copper-dependent enzymes are when copper bonds with enzymes (cuproenzymes), which can create energy, connective tissue, along with aiding in the central nervous system, with neurotransmitters and the myelin sheath formation and maintenance, forming melanin, and metabolizing iron.[181]

Possible Deficiency

- Anemia, birth defects, bleeding under skin, brittle bones, dermatitis, diarrhea, dilated veins, elevated cholesterol, hair loss, infections, lethargy, low body temperature, low white blood cell count, osteoporosis, pale skin pigmentation, sores, stunted growth, thyroid problems, uneven heartbeat
- Infants born prematurely, deficiency caused because copper isn't transferred until last of pregnancy.

Menkes' disease

- Fatal genetic disease of an abnormal copper metabolism.
- Children die about 2-3 years old.
- Kinky white hair.
- Brain cells die.
- Abnormal blood vessels, twisted and rupture.
- Weak bones.
- No cure.

Wilson's disease

- Can't get rid of excess copper.

- Accumulation in brain, eyes, liver, kidney.
- Needs to eat a copper-free diet.

Warnings, Precautions, and Side Effects

- Too much zinc can interfere with copper, ratio 10 parts zinc to 1 part copper.
- Toxic at 10 mg daily, so use in moderation.
- At 10 mg daily, may cause headaches, dizziness and vomiting.
- Poisons the liver, like jaundice, swelling of abdomen, signs like hepatitis.
- Behavioral disturbances, neurosis and psychosis.
- Neurological signs like Parkinson's disease and multiple sclerosis.
- Treatment for toxicity is penicillamine, a derivative of penicillin.
- High levels can cause heart and vascular disease.
- High levels can block selenium from performing its antioxidant duties.
- Copper deficiency can cause iron anemia.

Properties

- Analgesic, anti-arthritic, anti-ulcer, antibacterial, antimicrobial, antioxidant, pro-oxidant[182]

Food Sources

- Almonds, apricots, avocado, banana, barley, beans, beet roots, blackstrap molasses, broccoli, cashews, crab, chicken, cocoa, dandelion greens, dried peas and beans, fruit, garlic, halibut, lentils, liver, meat, mushrooms, navy beans, nuts, oats, oranges, organ *oysters, peanuts, pecans, radishes, raisins, salmon, seafood, sesame seeds, shellfish, soybeans, sunflower seeds, vegetables, walnuts, wheat bran, wheat germ, whole grain wheat

- Copper content is spent after being stored a while in cans.

Non-food Sources
- Copper cookware, copper plumbing, copper dishes
- Use copper bowl to beat egg whites and copper from bowl will go into the eggs.

Fluorine (Fl)

- Halogens element.
- Most reactive element.
- Caustic and very toxic gas.
- Attacks inert materials.
- Forms compounds with heavier noble gasses.

Fluoride   (F-)

- A negative ion of fluorine.
- It is a powerful enzyme poison.[183]

Two Types [184]

1. Natural occurring fluoride
   - Calcium-fluoride, when a calcium molecule connects to a fluoride molecule.
     - Easier for the fluoride to be absorbed into teeth.
     - Calcium-fluoride usually comes in a varnish that you paint on your teeth, the viscosity allows the fluoride to stay right where you want it until it is fully absorbed.
   - Not found to be toxic in any dose a human would consume.

2. Artificial fluoride made from aluminum by-products, manufactured by man.
   - Sodium fluoride and silica fluoride are aluminum waste bi-products.
   - Our water systems are treated with this fluoride.
   - Most dental products are made with foams, gels and rinses of this fluoride.
   - It can be absorbed under the tongue and into the soft gingiva (gums) where you don't want or need fluoride.
   - Controversy is whether it's toxic or not.
   - It is toxic in high doses.

Possible Uses
   - Dental disease, osteoporosis[185], rodent poison, strengthens bones and teeth

Possible Detriment
   - ADD/ADHD, birth defects, brittle bones with age, osteoporosis[186], rare bone cancer[187], thyroid dysfunction[188]

- Lowers Intelligence Quotient (IQ).[189]
- Alzheimer's disease is linked to fluoride and aluminum use.[190]
- Increase of hip fractures.[191]
- Crohn's disease bone loss has been treated with sodium fluoride but it was found to have no benefit over calcium and cholecalciferol.[192]

Warnings, Precautions, and Side Effects
- Do not use while pregnant or breastfeeding.
- According to Clinical Toxicology, 1984, fluoride is more noxious than lead, and slightly less noxious than arsenic.
- Green and black teas are magnets for fluoride.
- Interferes with mineralization of bones and teeth.
- Fluoride accumulates in the brain and body.
- Chelates calcium and iodine.
- Calcium fluoride added to water supply is a potent catalase poison.
- Fluorosis - when natural fluoride in water is high, a child's tooth enamel may become spotted.
- Debate whether artificial fluorination causes birth defects, bone deformities, cancer, and other health problems.
- Avoid if you have allergies, arthritis, bleeding, bone fragility, bursitis, diabetes, gall bladder maladies, heart problems, kidney problems, mental problems, and mental disturbances.
- Teflon and polytetrafluoroethylene are used in cookware, surgical implants, and reconstructive surgery.
- Fluoride based pesticides/fungicide, Cryolite and Sulfuryl fluoride, leach into our food supply, many times more concentrated than fluoridated tap water.
- Government doesn't require food labeling.

Food Sources
- Artificial fluoridation: prescription medications, salt, tap water, Teflon cookware (organofluorine compound), toothpaste
- Beer, citrus fruit, garlic, green and black tea, grape juice, land cress, potatoes, processed baby cereal, raisins, sage, soy, watercress
- Natural water, natural-occurring in fish, green and black tea (organically-grown has less fluoride), artificially-occurring fluoride tooth-paste

Research

The American Medical Association (AMA) published on December 8, 1993, a study associates a rare bone cancer to fluoride use, in which 27%-41% of women and men have hip breakage due to fluoridation.[193]

In a study of 202 postmenopausal women who have had osteoporosis and vertebral fractures, they found that the fluoride treated women had the bone density decrease by 4% and the nonvertebrae fractures were about three times higher, therefore it was not effective in treating osteoporosis.[194]

Germanium (Ge)

- Metalloids element.
- Recently discovered trace mineral by Japanese scientist, Kauhiko Asai.
- Dr. Asai believes all diseases are rooted by inadequate oxygen.
- Germanium attaches itself to oxygen molecules to improve molecular cell oxygenation, thus ridding body of toxins and poisons.

Possible Uses

- AIDS[195], angina pectoris[196], asthma[197], arthritis[198], atopic dermatitis, burn scaring, brain problems, cancer[199], candida and yeast infection, cataracts [200], chronic viral infections, depressive psychosis, edema, elevated cholesterol, empyema, eye problems, food allergies, HIV, heavy metal chelation(cadmium, mercury, other metal poisons)[201], hepatic dysfunctions[202], hepatitis[203], hepatoma, hypertension[204], intestinal cancer (natural organic germanium)[205], leukemia[206], liver cirrhosis, myocardial infarction [207], otitis media, progressive muscular atrophy (slows), Raynaud's disease[208], rheumatoid arthritis[209], senile osteoporosis[210], stress, tooth ache

Possible Benefits

- Increases oxygen in body.
- Introduction of interferon, macrophages, T-suppressor cells with natural killer cell activity.[211]
- Can facilitate high-energy electron energy.[212]

Properties

- Analgesia[213], anti-amyloidosis, anti-inflammatory[214], anticancer, antimicrobial[215], antioxidant, antitumor[216], antiviral[217], erythropoietin[218], free-radical scavenger[219], heavy metal detox[220], immune-enhancement[221], immunolomodulator, oxygen enrichment[222]

Food Sources

- Aloe Vera, comfrey, Cortinellus shiitake mushroom, garlic, grape wine, herb suma, kawaradake mushroom, mushrooms, onions, Siberian ginseng

Warning, Precautions, and Side Effects

- Chronic germanium intoxication was caused by way of supplementation, thus resulting in anemia, muscle atrophy, sensory impairment, tongue fasciculation, truncal ataxia, thus concluding in renal failure.[223]

Research

It's immunological and anti-viral properties induce interferon, macrophages and suppress T-cells while augmenting natural killer cells, which might be possible to treat or prevent AIDS.[224]

A 32 year old woman had Retro bulbar neuritis, blindness. Her vision had been declining for about a year. She was almost totally blind. She underwent the normal ophthalmic treatment without any success. The daughter rejected giving up so her father took her to the Organic Germanium Clinic although being doubtful for any success. Treatment began, she was given the mineral twice a day, orally, breakfast and supper, at the rate of 40 mg per I kg body weight. Within one month she could distinguish night and day. Her sight improved at 0.1in two months and 0.4 in several months and 1.0 in six months.[225]

Gold (Au)

- Transition Metal
- Chemically unreactive.
- Non-toxic internally or externally.
- Some claim it to have no known biological role.

Colloidal Gold

- Small microscopic gold particals suspended in water or another media.

Possible Uses
- Alzheimer's[226], anxiety, arthritis, brain lesions[227], bursitis, CNS inflammation[228], cancer immunodiangostics[229], cognitive function[230], depression, diabetes mellitus hepatic disease[231], diabetic insulin delivery[232], digestion, Parkinson's, rheumatism, rheumatoid arthritis[233], spinal cord injury[234], tendinitis

Possible Benefits
- Natural cell stimulant.
- Improves brain allertness, IQ concentration and memory.

Properties
- Anti-inflammatory[235], antibacterial, biomarker detection, germicidal, mood enhancer, nanoparticle drug delivery

Warning, Precautions, and Side Effects
- Excessive use can cause gold poisoning.

Food Sources
- Some mineral salts

Iodine   (I)

- Halogens element.
- Needed in trace amounts.
- Meat-eaters could be deficient.

Possible Uses

- Autism, brain damage[236], autoimmune thyroiditis[237], breast cancer[238], cognitive ability[239], colon cancer, defective neuromotor skills[240], defective speech/hearing[241], fibrocystic diseases, goiter, hair/nail/skin/teeth health, hyperthyroidism[242], mental development, mental retardation[243], metabolism, migraines, neuromuscular skills[244], physical development, prostate cancer[245], radio protective, slow pulse, subclinical hypothyroidism[246], thyroid health[247]

Possible Benefit

- Helps to metabolize excess fat.
- Sun-dried sea salt, Real salt or real Himalayan salt has iodine with the proper proportional 50-70+ trace mineral amounts required to give our body a synergistic effect.
- Essential component of the hormone thyroxin, which prevents goiter.
- The more iodine a diabetic takes, the less insulin required.
- For hypothyroid, the less thyroid medication needed.

Possible Deficiency

- Alopecia, anxious, clammy, decreased libido, dry hair, extremity coldness, increased weight, irritability, lethargy, low appetite, low energy production, lower body temperature, nervousness, obesity, thinning hair
- Unhealthy thyroid gland produces a goiter.
- "Betty Davis Eyes" - later symptom of hyperthyroidism.

* Brain damage caused by mother's low iodine causes birth defect of 10-15 IQ points lower.[248]

Test:

TPO Test - Thyroid Peroxidase Test shows and iodine and selenium deficiency.

The other Iodine non-Salt alternative
* Sea-vegetables like sea weed and kelp have natural iodine.
* Use liquid kelp in moderation.

Warnings, Precautions, and Side Effects
* Too much iodide, too little iodine can cause a goiter.
* Excess iodine (30x USDA) has a metallic taste, sores in the mouth, swollen salivary glands, diarrhea and vomiting.
* Excessive amounts of iodized refined common table salt can affect an individual with either high or low thyroid problems.
* Brussels sprouts, cabbage, cauliflower, kale, peaches, pears, spinach, and turnips block the uptake of iodine if eaten in large amounts.
* Iodine-131 is the bad iodine, caused by radiation. Vitamin C helps mitigate tissue damage.

Food Sources
* Asparagus, cayenne, cod liver oil, cranberry, dairy, dulse, *eggs, fish, garlic, Himalayan salt, iodized salt, kelp, lima beans, mushrooms, navy beans, organic yogurt, peppermint, Real salt, salt-water fish, sea salt, seafood, *sea vegetables (weed), sesame seeds, soybeans, spinach, strawberries, turnip greens, white deep-water fish

- Supplemental recommended amount of 150 mcg of iodine in a multi-vitamins, no more than 450 mcg of iodine each day.

Research

In 1990, one-third of the world's population was iodine deficient. Nine years later, 75% of the counties with the affected populations began iodizing salt. The deficiency quickly disappeared. Sometimes the iodized salt can cause elderly people to have hyperthyroidism, especially if they are taking a lot.[249]

Oral Potassium Iodide (50-100 mg.) protects the thyroid from radioactive iodine 131 only if taken within 2 hours before to 8 hours after iodine 131 intake has occurred but the protective effects are 40-80% with a iodine sufficient diet, with an iodine insufficient diet, it is only 15-65% absorbed.[250]

Recipes

Iodine Tincture
- 2 oz. quality kelp
- Place it into a quart jar
- 40% vodka 80-100 proof
- 60% water
- Steep, shake occasionally in Mason jar for about 2-3 weeks
- Strain and discard kelp
- Use 5+ drops in cup of water/juice as needed
- Store in dark, cool place for 20+ years

Iron (Fe)

- Transition metal element.

2 kinds of iron
  1. Heme iron - liver is best, sorry!
   - Beef, chicken, fish and other animal meats are easiest for our bodies to absorb.

  2. Non-heme iron - vegetables, grains, meats, and again, liver is still best.
    - Amino acids in meats and vitamin C, ascorbic acid, are indispensable and can double iron absorption or even more
    - Doesn't absorb as well.

Possible Uses
   - ADD/ADHD[251], anemia iron deficiency, candida[252], chemotherapy-related anemia[253], cold weather (body warmer), connective tissue biosynthesis, cough (ACE inhibitors)[254], fatigue[255], female problems, hair loss, insomnia, low thyroid[256], menstrual flow, mental development[257], mouth cracks, muscle function, normal growth and development, predialysis anemia[258], pregnancy[259], promotes growth, renal failure anemia, restless legs syndrome[260], skin tone, stress

Possible Benefits
   - Ferrous succinate is the best absorbed non-heme iron.
   - Many enzymes depend on iron.
   - Critical mineral for hemoglobin formation, oxygenates red blood cells.
   - Carries oxygen from one cell to another and removes carbon dioxide. Oxygenates the brain through the bloodstream.

- Guards against too much zinc and phosphorous.
- Iron and copper help form and modify collagen and elastin.
- Neurotransmitter synthesis.
- Essential to enzymes concerned with energy release, metabolizing cholesterol.
- Helps oxygen get to our cells and transports carbon dioxide out.
- Resides in red blood cells, needed for formation of hemoglobin and myoglobin.
- Supplementing 200 mg ferrous sulfate 3 times daily may greatly reduce symptoms of restless legs syndrome in the elderly.
- Helps athletes endurance by carrying oxygen to the muscles.
- Promotes protein metabolism.
- In healthy people, the intestines regulate iron absorption.
- Helps red blood cells carry energy-giving oxygen to all of our body .
- It affects brain cells, myelin and neurotransmitters.[261]
- Bacteria needs iron to stay alive and reproduce.[262]
- With tuberculosis and malaria, the body takes iron out of circulation by storing it in bone marrow, liver and other areas where the bacteria can't reach it.
- Take iron in between meals, with vitamin C for maximum absorption.
- To increase iron intake, use a newer cast iron skillet which gives more iron that an older one.
- Stainless steel cookware gives off a small amount of iron along with chromium which is very important in trace minerals.

Possible Deficiency
- Body tension, brittle hair, concentration problems, disruptive behavior, dizziness, fatigue, fearfulness, headaches, lethargic, lower IQ, memory problems, not observant, paleness, rapid heart rate, short attention span, shoulder stiffness, sleeping problems, slow motor development, swollen glossy or smooth tongue, unhappy, weakness, withdrawal.
- Pica, eating ashes, chalk, dirt, sticks, ice.
- Finger/toe nails have spoon-shaped or ridges running lengthwise.
- Affects immune response, body temperature.
- Affects concentration and learning diminished.
- Iron deficiency influences thyroid hormone synthesis and supplementation improves iodine assimilation.[263]
- Impacts brain functioning: attention functions, neurotransmitter degradation, neurotransmitter synthesis, organogenesis, post-partum depression, protein synthesis, spatial memory, among other.[264]
- Insufficient iron in pregnant woman have shorter pregnancies, inadequate weight, and are usually less physically fit.[265]
- Insufficient iron in pregnant woman may cause a premature delivery, lack of the placenta delivering receptors with limited iron to protect the fetus, thus resulting in low birth weight.[266]

Hemochromatosis - rare disease
- Excess build-up of iron in the tissues
- Bronze skin pigment
- Cirrhosis
- Diabetes
- Heart disorders

Properties
- 2-edged sword, when ill with bacteria, fungus, infection, microbes, or virus and the such, iron might not be good, there is a lot of debate on this topic in the scientific journals whether it's helpful or harmful.
- Antiviral, pro-infection[267], probacterial[268], promicrobial[269], transporter

Warnings, Precautions, and Side Effects
- Use in moderation. More is NOT better.
- Do not give iron formula to infants, iron loading has recently been proposed as causing Sudden Infant Death along with other recognized reasons.[270]
- Be careful of chewable iron, an overdose can kill a child.
- If anemic, use more iron with vitamin C. Make spaghetti sauce in an iron skillet.
- Strenuous exercise and stress depletes iron.
- If having infection and you use iron, check to see if you get better or worse.
- Don't eat more meat, but eat smaller portions, more often.
- Low tolerance symptoms are constipation, diarrhea, heartburn, nausea, and stomachache.
- Anemia symptoms are cognitive impairment, fatigue, headaches, heart palpitations, sore tongue, shortness of breath, or with exercise, one may have chest pain.
- Long-term aspirin use may cause stomach bleeding, leading to an iron deficiency so drink lots of water.
- Constant use of antacids lesson the stomach's acidity, in return, reducing iron absorption.
- Drinking large amounts of milk may produce anemia, which may encourage stomach irritation and bleeding.
- Too much iron can create free radicals, damage blood vessels and increase cholesterol.

• Do not take iron in a multi-vitamin supplement, has a tendency to bind with other ingredients.
• Do not take vitamin E with iron.
• Excessive amounts of vitamin E and zinc interfere with iron absorption.
• Heavy perspiration depletes iron.
• Excessive bleeding (menstrual) can lead to anemia.
• Excess tea and coffee drinking can cause to a deficiency.
• Men and pre-menopausal and menopausal women need less.
• Coffee, tea, soybeans, and whole grains reduce the amount of absorbable iron at one time.
• When the body has excess stores of iron, it increase the risk or cancer[271], so don't take too much, especially in supplements.
• Excessive iron intake or storage is associated with colorectal cancer.[272]
• Iron accumulating in the aging brain might cause oxidative-stress and increase the possibility of neurodegenerative diseases like Alzheimer's and Parkinson's disease.[273]
• Iron is vital to bacterial growth.[274]
• Iron should be withheld from invading bacteria, fungi, protozoa and neoplastic cells.[275]
• Excessive iron stores might lower the immune system and allow infectious organisms and cancer cells to grow adversely.[276]

Food Sources
- Almonds, apricots, avocado, beef, beets, blackstrap molasses, brewer's yeast, broccoli, Brussels sprouts, caviar, cherry juice, chickpeas, chlorophyll, clams, dandelion greens, dates, dried fruit, duck, dulse, eggs, endive, enriched breads, enriched cereals, fish, fortified ready-to-eat cereals, garlic, green leafy vegetables, kelp, kidney, kidney beans, lamb, leafy green vegetables, land cress, lentils, lima beans, liver, millet, nettle, navy beans, nuts, organ meats like liver and giblets, parsley, peaches, pears, pinto beans, poultry, prunes, pumpkin, rice bran, sesame seeds, soybean hulls, sunflower, and squash seed kernels, sardines, sesame seeds, shell fish, shrimp, soybeans, spinach, Swiss chard tomato puree, watercress, wheat bran and germ, white beans, whole grains, wild and eastern oysters
- Soybean hulls have a higher iron absorption than other foods
- Take iron with an enhancing vitamin C nutrient to increase the iron's absorption

Non-Food Sources
- Iron cookware increases iron food content up to 30 times.
- Cooking in a new iron skillet, especially with acidic foods, like tomatoes

Research
> In the Journal of Orthomolecular Medicine, 1988 issue, one should not take iron if they have a bacterial infection, because bacteria need iron to grow.[277]

Lithium   (Li)

- Alkali metal.

Possible Uses
- Alzheimer's[278], amyotrophic lateral sclerosis (ALS-Lou Gehrig's disease)[279], bipolar disorder[280], brain injury[281], cerebral ischemia[282], dementia[283], manic-depressive disorder, mental health problems, spinal cord injury[284]

Properties
- Anti-aging[285], neuroprotective[286]

Warning, Precautions and Side Effects
- Can cause kidney or liver damage.
- Can cause brain damage, diarrhea, edema, frequent urination, hypothyroidism, kidney disease, lethargy, liver disease, memory problems, mental confusion, nausea, slurred speech, staggering gait, tremors, vomiting, weight gain

Overdose
- Lithium overdose is common.
- See physician immediately.

Food Sources
- Blue corn, cooked vegetables, eggs, fish, kelp, meat, milk, mineral water, mushrooms, mustard, nightshade plants, pistachios, sardines, sugarcane

Research
Bipolar disorder is connected with a greater risk for dementia. Lithium usage for bipolar patients showed a lower prevalence of Alzheimer's disease crucial process pathogenesis.[287]

Magnesium   (Mg)

- Alkaline earth metals element.
- Heat sensitive mineral.

Possible Uses

- Alcoholic delirium tremens/hallucinosis[288], alcoholism[289], angina[290], anxiety disorders[291], arrhythmia[292], asthma[293], atherosclerosis[294], back and neck pain, blood clotting[295], blood pressure control[296], calms nervous system, cancer, cardiac disease[297], cardiomyopathy[298], chronic fatigue syndrome[299], chronic nephritis adult seizures[300], circulatory diseases, colorectal cancer[301], congestive heart failure[302], convulsions, coronary spasms[303], depression[304], diabetes (type 2)[305], diabetic seizures, eclampsia[306], emotional upset, epilepsy [307], eye twitches[308], fatigue[309], fibromyalgia[310], fluid retention, glaucoma[311], hair loss, hearing loss[312], heart attack damage, heart disease, heart spasms, hyperactivity, hyperlipidemia[313], hyperthyroidism[314], hypocalcaemia[315], hypomagnesaemia[316], hypertension[317], irregular heartbeat, irritability, ischemic heart disease[318], leg cramps, migraines[319], mitral valve prolapse[320], muscle control, muscle spasms, nervousness, newborn convulsions [321], noise-induced hearing loss[322], osteoporosis[323], , panic disorders, preeclampsia[324], protein synthesis, Raynaud's spastic vessels[325], relaxes blood vessels, skin aging, stress, stroke, swollen gums, tetanus [326], tremors, urinary tract infection, vasospastic angina[327], vertigo[328], weak muscles
- PMS symptoms of abdominal bloating, breast tenderness, swelling extremities, weight gain. [329]

Possible Benefits

- Part of fight or flight response.

- Magnesium malate (malic acid, potent chelator) binds with aluminum to flush it from the body.
- Major electrolyte with potassium, and regulates sodium and calcium.
- Hard water is usually magnesium rich.
- Take with dolomite and trace minerals.
- Involved in activating 30+ enzymes and hormonal actions.
- Blocks neuromuscular transmissions.
- Reduces acetylcholine released by motor nerve impulses.
- Needed by pituitary gland.
- Needed for bone and teeth formation.
- Aids the central nervous system, neuromuscular, and cardiovascular systems.
- Crucial to metabolism of fats and energy production.
- Aids in the metabolizing of carbohydrates and DNA production.
- Beneficial for people with asthma and bronchitis, lessens constriction of airways.
- A considerable amount of magnesium is lost when one sweats.
- Mineral baths permeates our body cells, in the spinal fluid, blood serum, and intracellular liquid.
- Activates the regulation and metabolizing of calcium.
- Brain's blood vessel tissue has double the concentration of magnesium than any other body tissue.

Electrolytes conduct the body's electrical currents through intracellular and extracellular fluid.

Possible Deficiency
- 80%-90% of the people in the U.S are not recognized as magnesium deficient.[330]
- A deficiency increases acetylcholine release and can change cardiac and skeletal muscles.

- Can cause cardiac arrest (diastole).[331]
- Aluminum gravitates to a magnesium deficient brain.
- Symptoms include chronic twitching, muscle irritability, tremors.
- Can come about by long-term use of diuretics, alcohol abuse, prolonged vomiting or diarrhea.
- Large amounts of calcium can also bring about a magnesium deficiency.
- If too little magnesium, it allows calcium and sodium, constricting agents, to flood cells and knot muscle tissue.
- During alcoholic withdrawal, one may experience hallucinations.
- Magnesium deficiency is frequently at the foundation of refractory potassium deficiency, adding more potassium can't correct this; the magnesium must be corrected first.
- Animals can suffer blood vessel dilation, diarrhea, edema, hair loss, kidney damage, sticky coat and super-excitability.

Sports Anemia

Adult sudden death is connected to hypertrophic cardiomyopathy (HCM), a thickened, enlarged heart or arrhythmia, an irregular rhythm of the heart, caused by magnesium deficiency.[332]

Magnesium Test or Possible Treatment

- RBC Minerals or more commonly called Elemental Analysis in Packed Erythrocytes. This test examines the levels of eight minerals and seven toxic heavy metals. The minerals this test analyzes from inside the red blood cell includes magnesium, manganese, molybdenum, potassium, selenium, vanadium and zinc.
- Calcium/magnesium ratio: 3/2 ratio.
- Can enhance magnesium's healing power by getting enough B-6.

Properties

- Anti-inflammatory, antibacterial, anticonvulsant[333], antidepressant[334], anxiolytic[335], calmative, vasodilation

Warnings, Precautions, and Side Effects

- Can cause diarrhea, nausea, vomiting.
- Overdose can cause cardiac arrhythmia, coma, drowsiness, muscle weakness, respiratory depression, thirst and death.
- Milk/dairy can deplete magnesium.
- Large amounts of calcium can aggravate magnesium deficiency.
- Use of alcohol, diuretics, diarrhea, fluoride, high zinc, high vitamin D reduce magnesium in the body.
- A lot of fats, cod liver oil, vitamin D and calcium lessen magnesium absorption.
- Fatty dieters need more magnesium.
- Oxalic acid foods like almonds, chard, cocoa, rhubarb, spinach and tea hinder magnesium absorption .
- Heart medication, digitalis, chemotherapy, antibiotics which can reduce magnesium.
- Deficiency can be induced by diuretics, water pills, which excrete magnesium and potassium.
- Magnesium exit's the body by way of the kidneys, check with physician previous to use, may cause renal damage.

Food Sources

- Alfalfa sprouts, almonds, apples, apricots, artichokes hearts, avocado, bananas, barley grass, beet greens, black beans, black-eyed peas, blackstrap molasses, *bovine brain (Caution: mad cow disease transference), brewer's yeast, brown rice, buckwheat, bulgur, *brazil nuts, *bran ready-to-eat cereal (100%), cashews, cayenne, chlorophyll vegetables, cocoa, coconut (fresh), collards, curry, dairy products, dandelion greens, dark chocolate, desiccated liver, dried apricots, *egg yolks, figs, fish, garlic, great northern beans, haddock, halibut, hard water rich in magnesium, hazelnuts, kelp, kidney, leafy green vegetables (raw), lima beans, liver, meat, millet, mixed nuts, mustard powder, navy beans, oat bran, okra, parsley, peaches, peanuts, pine nuts, Pollock, potato, *pumpkin and *squash seed kernels, raw nuts and seeds, red clover, rye, salmon, seafood, seeds, sesame seeds, shrimp, sockeye salmon, soybean, soybeans, spinach, Swiss chard, firm tofu with nigari, tourla, tuna, walleye, watercress, wheat bran, wheat germ (raw), white beans, wheat grass, whole grains, whole wheat

Research

41 patients were treated with magnesium sulfate, 15 of which was intravenously, in which the variant angina attacks terminated promptly. Mg sulfate was administered previously to several other patients and prevented an attack.[336]

Epsom Salt
Magnesium Sulfate Heptahydrate

- Well-known bath salt, hydrated magnesium sulfate crystals.
- Water soluble.
- Absorbed by the body externally.
- Softens the skin and relaxing sore muscles.
- Cosmetic and medicinal uses.

Possible Uses

- Acne[337], anesthesia[338], arthritis[339], asthma[340], bath salts, bee stings, blood clots, boils, blood pressure control, bruises, carbuncles, cerebral palsy prevention[341], child birth discomfort, chickenpox/hives/poison ivy itching, circulation, colds, concentration, congestion, constipation, delay labor, digestion, energy production, foot soak, flushes toxins, heartburn, hemorrhoids[342], inflammation, insomnia, joint soreness and stiffness, leather tanning, migraines, mordant dyeing, muscle control, muscle cramps, muscle pain, myocardial infarction[343], ophthalmic conditions (conjunctivitis)[344], osteoarthritis, periodontal disease[345], raccoon repellent, rose plants, skin ailments, skin scrub, smelly feet, splinter removal, sprains, stress, sunburn, vaginal infection[346], vaginal inflammation[347], wounds

Possible Benefits

- Made up of magnesium and sulfates mostly.
- Improves oxygen.
- Supports 325 enzymes.[348]
- Regulate body's enzymes.
- Regulating electrolytes to improve nerve function.
- Improves ability to use insulin in body.
- Raises serotonin level to decrease stress and lift the mood.
- Important for fats and energy production.
- Improves strength and stamina, promotes adenosine troposphere production.
- Regulates electrolytes and improves nerve functioning.
- Organizing electrical impulses.
- Produces serotonin, mood lifter and relaxation.

• Used externally, in which case small amounts are absorbed through the skin, Epsom salts detoxifies the body, relieves joint and muscle pain, softens the skin, has antiseptic properties, and eases digestive function.

Properties
• Bronchodilator (nebulizer), purgative

Warning, Precautions and Side Effects
• Can give you diarrhea.

Research
The Epsom Salt Industry Council informs the public that magnesium is the second most plentiful element in human cells. It is also the fourth most important positively charged ion in the body. It is a crucial component for body functions. It aids with electrical impulse transmission, elimination of natural toxins, and muscle control. When deficient, it can cause arthritis, digestive illnesses, joint pain, and stress-related disorders.[349]

Epson Salts Sulfates

Possible Uses
• Aches, boils, bruises, carbuncles, flu, rheumatoid arthritis, skin ailments, sprains, strains

Possible Benefits
• Essential for good health.
• Flushes toxins.
• Improve nutrient absorption.
• Forms brain tissue and joint proteins.
• Helps prevent and relieve migraine headaches.

Properties

- Anti-inflammatory, antiseptic, laxative

Warning, Precautions, and Side-effects

- Stress reduces magnesium levels in blood, thus increasing adrenaline production, magnesium binds with serotonin in the brain causing one to relax.
- Do not use if you have heart or kidney disease.
- May cause muscle weakness, cramps and heart abnormalities.
- Because it's high magnesium concentration, enemas and internal ingestion of Epsom salts can result in fatalities if used improperly or excessively.

Recipes

Childhood Epilepsy Folk Remedy

- 100-150 mg. magnesium citrate with baking soda
Some testimonials said just the baking soda worked.

Rosacea and Itching

- 1/4 c. Epson salt in warm water and sponge on

Epson Salt - Sea Salt Bath Soak

- 4 c. Epson salt
- 2 c. sea salt
- Add 20+ drops essential oil: eucalyptus (sick), frankincense, lavender, lemon, mint, rose, etc.
- Mix and let dry
- Use 1 c. mixture each bath.

PMS Fluid Retention Symptom Reduction[350]

- 200 mg magnesium daily for 2 months
- First month has no effect. Second month does.

Manganese   (Mn)
Manganese superoxide dismutase (MnSOD)

- Alkaline earth metals element.

Possible Uses

- Alzheimer's[351], basal ganglia lesions[352], bladder cancer[353], blood sugar control, bone formation[354], brain function[355], breast cancer[356], cardiomyopathy[357], cardiovascular disease[358], cerebral reperfusion injury[359], colon cancer, colorectal cancer[360], connective-tissue[361], diabetes[362], digestion, epilepsy[363], female problems, headaches, inflammation[364], ischemic brain injury[365], menstruation, mitochondrial-related epileptic seizures, moods, nervous disorders, neurodegenerative disease[366], osteoporosis, pain, Parkinson's, post-menopause, seizure disorders[367], sex hormones, skin aging[368]

Possible Benefits

- Acts as a co-enzyme.
- Builds connective tissue.
- Helps with metabolizing amino acids, carbohydrates, cholesterol and fats.
- Increases mineral density of spinal bone.
- Helps to metabolize vitamin B-1 and E.
- Helps with the nervous system.
- MnSOD is an enzyme that repairs DNA.
- MnSOD protects against mitochondrial superoxide radical damage.
- MnSOD converts radicals into hydrogen peroxide H_2O_2 for reduction into water.
- MnSOD acts as an antioxidant, is found in the body's mitochondria where it provides protection against damage from free radicals during energy production.

• MnSOD protects the energy-generating mitochondria, and is the cells first defense against free radical damage.

Possible Deficiency
• Absentminded, bone and joint abnormalities, bone malformation, dizzy, growth retardation, hearing problems, heart problems, high blood pressure, high cholesterol, memory loss, muscular contractions, poor eyesight, shivers, tremors

Deficiency because of calcium/iron
• Cramping, eye problems, fast heartbeat, infertility, weakness

Properties
• Anti-inflammatory, anticancer[369], antioxidant, antitumor[370] , inflammatory cytokine[371]

Warnings, Precautions, and Side Effects
• High concentrations are toxic to cells.
• MnSOD has been associated with prostate cancer development.[372]

Overdose Toxicity
• Can cause liver damage, muscle spasms.
• Excessive CNS storage looks like idiopathic Parkinson's disease.[373]
• Environmental manganese dust absorbed by miners is very toxic, can cause psychiatric problems, respiratory inflammation, and organic brain disease.

Food Sources

- *Almonds, avocados, banana, beetroot, blackberries, blueberries, *brown rice, buckwheat, carrots, cereal, chestnut, cloves, *coconut, cucumber, dried beans and peas, egg yolks, figs, fruits, and peas, garlic, ginger, grapes, green beans, *green leafy vegetables, hazelnuts, kiwi, land cress, legumes, lettuce, liver, molasses, mustard greens, nettle, nuts, oats, organ meats, peas, peppermint, pineapple, raspberries, red clover, seaweed, seeds, spinach, strawberries, tea leaves, tofu, tropical fruits, turmeric, watercress, whole grains, whole wheat

Molybdenum   (Mo)
Aldehyde oxidase   Xanthine oxidase

• One of the most complex of Transitional metals elements.

Possible Uses
   • Aches and pain, anemia[374], asthma, blood sugar control[375], bone health, colon cancer[376], colorectal cancer[377], dental care[378], diabetes[379], esophagus cancer[380], mouth and gum microwave disorders[381], pancreatic cancer[382], post ischemic cardiac function[383], sexual impotence in older men[384]

Possible Benefits
   • Use with copper for movement.
   • Aids enzymes and helps metabolizes amino acids.
   • Cofactor enzymes concerned in protein synthesis.
   • Essential nutrient enables body to release iron for oxygen.
   • Required by enzymes to use carbon, sulfur and nitrogen.
   • Essential for all body functions.
   • Reduces ammonia.
   • Involved as part of the enzyme system, aiding with metabolizing carbohydrates, fats, and protein.
   • More molybdenum reduces allergic reactions to sulfites.
   • People with Wilson disease can be treated with molybdenum to counteract too much copper, although zinc can treat it better at lower levels.

Properties
   • Antidiabetic[385], antioxidant, antiproliferative[386], antitumor[387], cytotoxic[388]

Warnings, Precautions, and Side Effects
* People with little molybdenum show more signs of allergies to sulfites, asthma-type symptoms that may cause an allergic reaction resulting in death.
* Too much molybdenum can prompt gout-like symptoms.
* High intake of sulfur can lessen molybdenum.
* Too much molybdenum can interfere with copper.
* Enzymes may contribute to neurological disorders like alcohol liver injury, Amyotrophic lateral sclerosis (ALS – Lou Gehrig's disease), Parkinson's, schizophrenia and visual problems.[389]

Food Sources
* Barley, beef liver, beans, buckwheat, cauliflower, cereal grains, dark leafy green vegetables, dried peas, green beans, green leafy vegetables, legumes, lentils, lima beans, liver, meat, organ meats, peas, soybeans, spinach, sunflower seeds, wheat germ, whole grains

Non-food Sources
* May be found in steel and cast iron pans.

Phosphorus   (P)

- Nonmetal element.
- 2nd most abundant mineral in body and works with calcium.
- Most important element in healthy soil.

Possible Uses
- Alcoholism, arthritis, bone and tooth formation, bone mass[390], brain functioning, Celiac disease, Crohn's, digestion, energy, heart muscle contraction, hormone balance, hypophosphate (low phosphorus)[391], hypercalcemia (high calcium)[392], osteoporosis[393], pyorrhea, tooth decay[394], weakness

Phosphorus-32 Possible Uses
- Radioisotope has 14.3 day half-life, emits beta-rays.
- Used in Sodium phosphate (P-32) form.
- Chronic lymphocytic leukemia, chronic myelocytic leukemia, polycythemia vera.

Possible Benefits
- Keep calcium and phosphorus in balance.
- Helps the body utilize and balance vitamins, including D and the minerals iodine, magnesium, and zinc.
- Used for the brain, blood, heart, and kidney.
- Aids with cell growth, repair and chemical reactions.
- Energy extraction to different parts of the body.
- Aids in cell and tissue repair and protein formation.
- Needed for the genetic building blocks of DNA and RNA.
- Excreting wastes from kidney.
- Essential to assimilate body fat.
- Calcium, magnesium, and phosphorus, needed in correct balance, with surplus or inadequate amounts, bad effects can result.

- Calcium: phosphorus ratio is 2.5:1

Possible Deficiency
- Anxiety, appetite loss, bone problems, fatigue, irregular breathing, joint problems, numbness, constrained growth, rickets, skin sensitivity, stamina, stressed, tooth decay, tremors, weak bones, weight loss

Calcium, Phosphorus and Magnesium Deficiency[395]
- Involves bone, intestines, and kidney.
- People who have hypocalcaemia (low calcium), hypophosphate (low phosphate), and hypomagnesaemia (low magnesium) have low gastrointestinal assimilation.
- Hyperphosphatemia (too much phosphates) and hypomagnesaemia (too much magnesium) can cause kidney disease.

Warning, Precautions and Side Effects
- See your health care provider if using alcohol, medications or diuretics.
- Can be toxic and cause diarrhea, calcification or hardening of internal organs, or can interfere with mineral absorption.
- Phosphorus must be balanced with calcium.
- Antacids deplete phosphorus.
- Too much phosphorus is associated with cardiovascular disease and kidney disease.
- Renal Secondary Hyperparathyroidism is where the kidney fails and at getting rid of surplus phosphorus.[396]

Food Sources

• Alfalfa, asparagus, bone meal, bran, brewer's yeast, broccoli, cayenne, corn, dairy products, dandelion greens, dried fruit, eggs, fish, garlic, legumes, meat, nuts, *peanut butter, peas, potato, pumpkin seeds, meats, nuts, peanut butter, *pork, poultry, rice, sage, salmon, sesame seeds, sunflower seeds, *tuna, watercress, wheat germ, white bread, whole grains

• Soda pop carbonated beverages are high in phosphorus but an excessive amount can cause undesirable side effects.

Article

In the article by Sally Squires, "The Amazing Statistics and Dangers of Soda Pop," she explains that soda pop is the beverage of choice, leading to caffeine dependence, obesity, tooth decay and weakened bones. The overload of phosphorus is depleting calcium from the bones, making them weaker and prone to fracture.[397]

Potassium   (K)

- Alkali metals element.
- Critical to life.

Possible Uses

- Acute myocardial infarction[398], alkalosis associated with potassium deficiency[399], apathy[400], asthma[401], blood pressure control[402], body energizer, cardiovascular[403], chronic illness, chronic obstructive pulmonary disease (COPD) [404], constipation, depression, diabetes[405], early childhood intractable epilepsy[406], exhaustion, fatigue, flabby muscles, heart failure[407], heat exhaustion, heat stroke[408], hypertension[409], hypotension[410], insomnia, irritable[411], ischemic heart disease[412], listlessness, lymphocytic leukemia[413], malnutrition[414], multiple sclerosis[415], muscle health, muscle relaxation[416], muscular dystrophy[417], nerve health, nervous system, old age weakness[418], rheumatoid arthritis[419], skin care, slow heartbeat, stroke prevention[420], underweight

Possible Benefits

- Maintains water balance, necessary for digestion.
- Necessary for tissue formation.
- Helps in the stability of some enzymes.
- Red blood cells need potassium.
- Corrects acid-base (pH) balance and electrolyte balance.
- Essential for older adults who have low blood pressure.
- Crucial for nerve conduction, muscle message transmission, carbohydrate, glucose, protein metabolization.

• Pushes sodium out of the body, some salt substitutes have potassium chloride and the chloride may entice the body to hold on to its sodium (people with kidney disease may want to keep away from salt substitutes, check with physician).

• Released through diarrhea, sweating, urination, and vomiting.

• Potassium-to-sodium ratio should be 5:1, so if you're eating a lot of sodium (salt), white common table salt…stops it.

Potassium-Salt Balance

• Regulates some muscles.
• Regulates some nerve functions.
• Transfers fluids from cells and bloodstream to create homeostasis.
• Too much salt blocks potassium health benefits, therefore increasing blood pressure.

Possible Deficiency

• Rare
• Uncontrolled diabetes.
• Important mineral to reload upon after intense exercise.
• Happens to people who are taking diuretics.
• People with prolonged water loss.
• Early signs are muscle weakness, confusion, falling blood pressure, irritability, slow reflexes, and fatigue.
• Depletion leads to abnormal heart rhythm, into a heart attack, then death.
• Hormonal therapies like aldosterone, cortisone, DCA, etc.
• In adolescents, it's acne and in mature adults, it's dry, sagging skin.
• Muscular degeneration.

• Severely protein malnourished people may have very little potassium in their brain, which can cause apathy, irritability, stupor, coma, and then death.[421]

• People tend to overload on sodium which depletes potassium, thus increasing the likelihood of cardiovascular disease.

Warnings, Precautions, and Side Effects

• Licorice decreases potassium.

• Chronic illness, diarrhea, extensive surgeries, malnutrition, sweating, vomiting can cause deficiency.

• Too much can cause arrhythmias.

• Diuretics, diarrhea, laxatives and kidney disorder interfere with potassium levels.

• In diabetic patients, where potassium is low, fruit juice or broth is given to prevent coma.

• People with heart conditions should be aware of sun/heat problems because potassium evacuates the body quickly.

Food Sources

• *Apples, apricots, avocados, *bananas, beans, beet greens, blackstrap molasses (1 T), bok choy, brewer's yeast, broccoli, brown rice, Brussel sprouts, buttermilk, cantaloupe, carrots, cauliflower, clams, cod, dairy foods, dandelion greens, dates, desiccated liver, *dulse, figs, dried fruit, *fish, fruit, garlic, halibut, honeydew melon, ketchup, legumes, lentils, lima beans, *meat, melons, *milk, nuts, oranges, organ meat, parsley, peaches, pork, potato with skin, poultry, prunes, rainbow trout, rockfish, seeds, soybeans, spinach, squash, sunflower seeds, sweet potato, tomato, tourla, tuna, vegetables, watercress, wheat bran, wheat germ, white beans, whole grains, winter squash, yams, yogurt, plain and non-fat

Research

Thirty-six children with epilepsy resilient to traditional treatment were given potassium bromides with the present therapy. 13 children received no benefit from this procedure. Nine achieved a 50% reduction and nine children became seizure-free. Those who had tonic and focal seizures had no reaction. Only about one-third experienced side effects but was declared as tolerable. The daily dosage range was 50-80 mg. potassium bromide per kg body weight. A favored indication of bromides for early onset epilepsy patients with generalized tonic-clonic seizures and/or alternating hemi-grand mal, to which other treatments are unsuccessful.[422]

Recipe

Dr. Chase's Recipes   1881   Asthma Tea [423]

Iodide of potassium has a bad case of Asthma, by taking 5 gr. Doses, 3 times daily. Take 1/2 oz. and put it into a vial, and add 32 tea-spoons of water-then 1 tea-spoon of it will contain the 5 grs., which put into 1/2 gill more of water, and drink before meals.
* A gill is 1/4 of a pint.

Selenium   (Se)

- Nonmetal element.
- An absolutely essential micronutrient, we die without it.
- Selenium availability depends upon the amount of sulfur and sulfur-containing amino acids to for enzyme glutathione peroxidase.
- Super Star of mineral antioxidants, and functions as an antioxidant, and is part of enzyme glutathione peroxidase.
  - Which helps protect against oxidative damage.
  - Constituent of blood platelets and white blood cells.

Possible Uses

- AIDS[424], Alzheimer's sporadic dementia[425], anemia, bladder cancer[426], bone marrow cisplatin nephrotoxicity[427], breast cancer[428], cancer[429], candida[430], cardiomyopathy[431], cardiovascular disease[432], cataracts[433], cirrhosis[434], cognitive decline[435], colon cancer[436], colorectal cancer[437], congestive heart disease, Cystic Fibrosis[438], dandruff shampoo, epilepsy[439], eye diseases, fatty liver syndrome, flu lung infections[440], fetus brain development[441], gastrointestinal cancer[442], hepatitis B[443], hepatitis[444], hepatitis C virus-induced liver cancer[445], Hodgkin's disease[446], human leukemia[447], immune system, inflammation, intestinal cancer[448], ischemic heart disease[449], Keshan disease[450], kwashiorkor[451], liver cancer[452], lung cancer[453], mercury toxicity, metal chelation, muscles, muscular dystrophy [454], myocarditis[455], Parkinson's[456], prenatal infant growth, prostate cancer[457], rheumatoid arthritis[458], serious forms of psoriasis[459], skeletal muscle pain, skin cancer prevention, stomach cancer[460], stroke[461], sudden infant death syndrome (SIDS)[462], UV light radiation[463]

Possible Benefit
- May prevent malignant cell replication.
- Prevents free radical cell damage.
- Assists white blood cells.
- Most effective when taken with vitamins A and E.
- Can help thwart skin cancer.
- It can replace sulfur in proteins.
- Needed for pancreatic function.
- Aids in tissue elasticity.
- Helps the body absorb vitamin antioxidants.
- Concentrated in kidneys, liver, pancreas, spleen, and testicles.
- Helps make the thyroid hormone.
- Seaweed contains both iodine and selenium and in Japan where it is a popular, breast cancer is less than in the US.
- Iodine plus selenium works better at reducing benign breast disease and thyroid, goiter, a potent anti-cancer antioxidant combination.
- Fortifies the immune system, reduces the rate of cancer in humans and helps to alleviate leukopenia, (abnormal decreases of white blood cells).

Possible Deficiency
- Anemia, inflammation, high blood pressure, cardiac dysfunction, premature aging, and reduced male sex potency.
- Linked to cancer, poor blood clotting, sudden death, and controversy over heart disease.
- Breakdown of muscles, including the heart.
- Abnormalities in brain, genital tract, heart, liver, pancreas, striated muscle.[464]
- Deficiency increases viral infection risks. [465]

Properties

- Anti-angiogenesis[466], anti-inflammatory, antibacterial, anticancer[467], anticarcinogenic, antifungal, antineoplastic[468], antioxidant[469], antitumor[470], antiviral[471], apoptosis[472], cell proliferation[473], chemo preventive[474]

Warnings, Precautions, and Side Effects

- Can be toxic in supplement form.
- Do not take selenium for preventing cardiovascular disease.[475]
- Mercury blocks selenium, so some ocean fish might not be good.
- Extremities nerve problems, fatigue, hair loss, nail changes, nausea, vomiting.
- May cause depression nausea, nervousness, vomiting.
- Lack of selenium during pregnancy may contribute to Muscular Dystrophy in the baby.[476] It's also important for the mother to have adequate selenium when breastfeeding.
- Overdose may cause selenium-induced cataracts.[477]
- Selenium supplements aren't endorsed for cardiovascular disease.[478]

Food Sources

- Beans, *brazil nuts, brewer's yeast, broccoli, brown rice, cabbage, chicken, corn, dairy products, egg yolks, fish, garlic, kidneys, liver, molasses, oats, ocean fish, onion, red grapes, rice, salmon, seafood, seaweed, selenomethionine (nutritional yeast with high selenium), tourla, *tuna fish, vegetables, wheat germ, whole wheat, whole grains

* Best of the rest

Tuna

Brazil nut is also rich and you only need a few nuts a day.

Selenium, oltipraz, vitamin C and flavones are agents that block or suppress mutation.[479]

Concerning the family of genes, BRCA, this is involved in mending damaged genes. Mutations hinder it from working properly. When this happens, it multiplies the breast cancer risk fracture. Research in Cancer Epidemiology discovered that if one were to supplement 690 mg of selenium, twice daily, it healed the gene damage rate with BRCA1 mutations. They found this research short but encouraging.[480]

Silicon　(Si)
Silica　　Silanate　　Silicic acid

- Metalloids element.
- More vital than iron, needed for daily consumption.

Possible Uses

- Alopecia (hair loss)[481], atherosclerosis[482], bone density[483], bone formation[484], breast implants, brittle hair, brittle nails, cardiovascular disease[485], degenerative diseases[486], filtering waste, hair/nails/skin care, insomnia, osteoporosis[487], premenopausal bone density[488], sprains, strains, tuberculosis[489], water treatment

Possible Benefits

- Essential for growth.
- Helps maintain connective tissue and healthy arteries.[490]
- Restores calcium/magnesium balance.
- Necessary to assimilate phosphorous.
- Boron, calcium, magnesium, manganese and potassium help utilize silicon efficiently.

Possible Detriment

- There has been a great debate over decades as to whether silicone breast implants cause Connective Tissue Disease to which, they didn't find any conclusive evidence.[491]

Possible Deficiency

- Aging skin, bone deformities, brittle nails, thinning hair, wrinkles

Warnings, Precautions, and Side Effects
- Do not use if pregnant or breast feeding.
- May cause hives, itching, rashes, difficulty breathing, tightness, excessive burning, redness, stinging, peeling, tender skin.
- Doesn't help post-menopausal bone density.[492]
- Do not use if you have chronic kidney disease.
- Aluminum and silicon (aluminosilicates) are at the center of neurofibrillary tangles in Alzheimer's disease.[493]

Food Sources
- Alfalfa, almonds, apples, barley, beets, bell peppers, brown rice, carrots, cereals, cucumber, dandelion greens, fish, honey, horsetail grass (herb), leafy green vegetables, legumes, mother's milk, oats, onions, oranges, parsley, peanuts, pumpkins, soybeans, spinach, raw cabbage, unrefined grains, watercress, whole grains

Research

Silicon is extremely important for connective tissue functioning, especially in the cartilage and bone, with the organic matrix. It is also the key ion in the active state of estrogenic cells. It also acts in the subcellular enzyme-containing structures biochemistry.[494]

Silver   (Ag)

- Transition metals element.
- Silver is considered to be non-toxic.
- Strong inorganic compound.

Historical Perspective

- For thousands of years, it has been used as a natural antibiotic.
- During Europe's 14th century black plague bacterium epidemic, the wealthy didn't get the illness. The assumption was that they were protected by using silverware and silver pacifiers.
- Earlier pioneers placed silver dollars in milk to keep it fresh.
- In the late 1800s, Carl Sigmund Franz Credé, a German obstetrician discovered how to prevent newborn infant ophthalmic neonatorum eye blindness by using silver nitrate. (Credé Silver Method)
- In 1917, Dr. Malcolm Morris reported to the British Medical Journal that silver "…has a distinctly soothing effect. It rapidly subdues inflammation and promotes healing of the lesions; it can be used with remarkable results in enlarged prostate with irritation of the bladder, in pruritis ani and perineal eczema, and in hemorrhoids."
- In World War II, Dr. Charles Fox battled bacterial wound infections with silver sulfadiazine.
- Dr. Margraf diluted silver nitrate and found that it destroys Pseudomonas aeruginosa bacterium in burn cases and skin ulcers for faster healing, but found it to disturb the body salt balance and wasn't as feasible.

• In the 1990's the Chinese government began researching silver to develop a powerful antiseptic. Their research helped develop a silver-based compound that could sterilize surfaces for extensive periods of time without causing any toxic reactions to humans.

• The FDA approves a few uses of silver for medical use, such as silver sulfadiazine, sold under the name Silvadene, which is used to protect burns from bacterial infections in many hospitals.

Possible Uses

• AIDS[495], allergies[496], Alzheimer's detection[497], appendicitis[498], asthma[499], athlete's foot[500], Bacillus subtilis[501], bladder infection[502], blood parasites[503], blood poisoning[504], boils[505], bone growth[506], bone reconstructive surgery[507], breast cancer[508], bronchial issues[509], bronchitis[510], bronchial asthma, bubonic plague[511], burn treatment[512], cancer therapy[513], candida albicans[514], candida globata[515], cervical cancer[516], chlamydia[517], cholera[518], chronic obstructive pulmonary disease[519], colitis[520], colorectal cancer[521], conjunctivitis[522], coronavirus[523], cystitis[524], dermatitis[525], dental plaque[526], diabetes[527], diabetic skin ulcer[528], diarrhea, dysentery[529], E coli[530], ear infection[531], eczema[532], enteric fever[533], epiglonitis[534], eye infection[535], fibrositis[536], food poisoning[537], Gardnerella Vaginitis[538], gastritis[539], gonorrhea[540], grafting[541], gram-negative[542], gram-positive bacteria[543], HIV-1[544], hay fever[545], hepatitis B virus[546], herpes[547], hypertrophy scar formation[548], immune system boost, impetigo[549], indigestion, infections[550], itching, keratitis[551], laryngitis, Legionnaire's disease silver-based water purifying systems[552], leprosy[553], leukemia[554], lung disease[555], lupus[556], lymphangitis[557], Lyme disease[558], MRSE[559], malaria[560], male reproduction[561], meningitis[562], methicillin-resistant Staphylococcus aureus (MRSA)[563],

Neisseria gonorrhea[564], neurasthenia[565], osteomyelitis[566], parasites[567], Parkinson's[568], pathogenic viruses[569], pleurisy[570], pneumonia[571], post-surgical infection[572], prostate cancer[573], psoriasis[574], purulent ophthalmia[575], respiratory tract infection (nose, sinus, larynx), rhinitis[576], rheumatism[577], ringworm[578], Salmonella typhus[579], scarlet fever[580], septic conditions[581], severe acute respiratory syndrome (SARS)[582], shingles[583], sinus infection[584], skin cancer[585], sore throat[586], staph infections[587], strep infections[588], Streptococcus pyogenes[589], stomach ulcers[590], syphilis[591], throat infection[592], thyroid[593], tooth decay[594], toxemia[595], trachoma[596], trench foot[597], tuberculosis[598], ulcers[599], urinary tract infection[600], viral and fungal parasites[601], water treatment, whooping cough[602], wood preservation, wound healing[603], yeast infections[604]

Possible Benefits

- Silver kills 650 disease organisms.[605]
- Silver interrupts proper oxygen processing by an enzyme.
- Bacteria die without oxygen.
- 90% of US burn centers use silver.
- Used in artificial transplants.[606]
- Used in new-age drugs.[607]
- Topical stem cell activation.[608]
- Fights antibiotic resistant bacteria.[609]
- Used for antibiotic delivery as well as in gene delivery system.[610]
- Structural changes happen in cell membrane when small particles of silver and sulfur combine.[611]
- Silver is utilized in many ways, as nanoparticles, silver ions or salt, silver nitrate, silver sulfadiazine, silver-based compounds, Nano gels, nana lotions, also silver coating on silver devices.

Properties
- Antibacterial[612], antibiotic[613], antifungal[614], antiseptic, antimicrobial[615], antiviral[616], bactericidal[617], broad-spectrum antimicrobial[618], cytotoxic, cytoprotective[619], genotoxic[620], immunomodulating[621]

- Silver nanoparticles are atomic size particles, extremely small. Metallic nanoparticles are considered the best antibacterial agents.[622]

Warning, Precautions and Side Effects
- Mining silver can get into the lungs and get argyria (bluish-grayish-black skin color).
- Inhaled silver can become lung infection and change into Sprague-Dawley.[623]

True Colloidal Silver

- Solution of microscopic ultra-fine particles of silver suspended in water.[624]
- Electrical silver atoms.
  - True colloidal silver has no taste, extremely high atomic size silver particle concentration, in parts per million, and requires no refrigeration.

Possible Uses
One-cell bacteria[625], fungi[626], infections[627], viruses[628] and more, see silver above.

Warnings, Precautions, and Side effects

- CNN and Consumer Report have warned of the dangers from taking colloidal silver. Each organization failed to research easily obtainable information about the possible cause of argyria. Contrary to the reports issued by these two organizations, true colloidal silver is not the cause of argyria. Products that have been known to lead to argyria are solutions of silver protein and solutions of silver ions; neither of these products are true colloidal silver.[629]
- Must be taken responsibly in moderation.
- Might cause toxicity in large amounts.
- Manufacturers of true colloidal silver have warned of the risk associated with making solutions of silver protein and solutions of silver ions from kits for years. To learn about the nature of many of the more common silver products go to:

http://www.silver-colloids.com/Reports/reports.html
Pay particular attention to the classification as either 1) true colloidal silver, 2) ionic silver or 3) silver protein.
- Ionic silver is extremely volatile and may bond with chloride in your body, turning into a useless compound.
- Silver protein can cause argyria.

Research

1-10nm silver nanoparticles can attach and inhibit the HIV-1 virus from binding with host cells.[630]

Dr. Richard L. Davies, Executive Director of the Silver Institute, which monitors silver technology in 37 nations, reports, "In four years we've described 87 important new medical uses for silver. We're just beginning to see to what extent silver can help promote healthy body function."[631]

Colloidal Silver	**Antibiotics**
Doesn't suppress immune system.	Suppresses immune system.
Helps combat vitamin deficiencies.	Can cause a vitamin deficiency.
Only kills harmful pathogens.	Inhibit the growth of bad disease-causing bacteria.
Doesn't hurt helpful essential "friendly" bacteria in the digestive system.	Destroys helpful essential bacteria in the digestive system.
	Can cause diarrhea.
Doesn't create "super bugs."	Can create "super bugs." Antibiotics kill 95% of harmful pathogens but 5% opposes the antibiotics and live.
Resistant-strains don't develop.	Resistant-strains can develop.

Sodium (Na)

- Alkali metals element.
- Essential in small amounts.

Possible Uses
- Adrenal insufficiency (Addison's disease)[632], blood pressure regulation[633], confusion, dehydration, diarrhea, dizziness, excessive perspiration, glucose (sugar) absorption[634], heart palpitation, heat muscle cramps[635], lethargy, low blood pressure, muscle cramps, nervous system, sunstroke, vomiting, weakness

USDA Recommended Daily Allowance
- 1 teaspoon or 2.4 grams
- This is total consumption of all salts, what is included in the foods, drinks and shaken from the salt shaker.

Possible Benefit
- Heat resistant.
- Regulates water.
- Regulates blood pressure, blood volume, equilibrium, muscles and nerve impulses.
- Sugar assimilation is dependent upon salt.[636]
- Maintains a proper water balance and blood pH.
- Needed for muscle, nerve, and stomach function.
- If you take a lot of sodium, you need more potassium.
- Eliminates excess carbon dioxide.
- Maintains acid-base alkali phosphates balance.
- A positive charged ion, having too much or too little can cause an electrolyte imbalance.

Electrolytes conduct the body's electrical currents through intracellular and extracellular fluid.

Warnings, Precautions, and Side Effects
- Too much salt informs the kidneys to restrain water.
- Too little salt permits kidneys to evacuate water.
- Too much salt can cause weight gain by way of salty fast foods, or water retention.
- Manufactured foods are often higher in sodium chloride to help process and preserve the food as well as make it taste better. Check the contents on the back of the product for sodium amount.
- Unbalanced salt/potassium intake can lead to heart disease.
- Excess salt might cause edema, heart attack, high blood pressure, hypertension, liver and kidney disease, potassium deficiency, stomach cancer, stroke, vascular diseases.
- Do not use or use sparingly if you have edema or kidney problems.
- Ordinary common table salt (sodium chloride) is said to be the cause of hypertension.
- Hyperuricemia can bring about salt sensitivity, initiating vascular disease.[637]
- Obesity can bring about a blood pressure rise resulting from salt sensitivity.[638]

Sodium Toxicity
- Cerebral edema, decreased urine output, dehydration, diarrhea, high blood pressure, low grade fever, muscle twitching, seizures, swelling of brain nerves, vomiting, can lead to coma

Insufficient Sodium
- Confusion, dry mucous membranes, edema, excessive blood loss, excessive fluid loss, excessive perspiration, headaches, hypotension, impaired kidney function, lethargy, muscle weakness. nausea, water intoxication, weak pulse, weight gain

Food Sources
- Almost all foods in varying degrees.
- Apples, baking soda, baking powder, bananas, biscuits, bread, butter, cabbage, carrots, celery, common table salt, dried peas, egg yolks, ham, leafy green vegetables, pickled foods, processed cheese, pulses, salty meats, sauces, sausage, smoked fish, snacks, turnips

Strontium   (Sr)
Strontium carbonate   strontium gluconate
strontium lactate
Strontium Ranelate (semi-synthetic patiented)

- Alkaline earth metal.
- Usually we hear only about the "bad" Strontium 90, the radioactive nuclear fallout isotope, which gets into the food-chain and can cause bone cancer and leukemia from extended exposure.
- But here is where I am writing about the "good" strontium.

Possible Uses

- Bone fracture prevention[639], bone growth, bone mineralization, bone tissue engineering[640], estrogen-related bone loss[641], hip fractures, metastatic bone cancer pain hot spots[642], osteopenia, osteoporosis[643], postmenopausal women bone health[644], vertebral fractures[645]

Possible Benefits

- Increases bone mass and bone formation.[646]
- Breaks down old bone to form new bone.
- Similar structure to calcium and helps pull calcium into the bones, enhances osteoblast, and aids cell building.
- Strontium carbonate nanoparticles (SCNs) are currently being tested as an anticancer drug delivery system.[647]
- Aids cell proliferation rate of human mesenchymal stem cells in bone formation and repair.[648]
- Used as a biodegradable, almost nontoxic, antitumor drug delivery system.[649]

Properties

- Anabolic, antioxidant, antiresorptive[650]

Warning, Precautions and Side Effects
- Supplements may have side effects like abdominal spasms, diarrhea, difficulty breathing, gas upsets, headaches, and memory problems.
- Consult physician if you have blood clots or kidney problems.
- Low calcium and magnesium with high strontium can cause bone deformities.

Food Sources
- Barley, beans, Brazil nuts, brown rice, carrots, celery, corn, dairy, leafy vegetables, legumes, lettuce, milk, mollusks, oysters, peas, potato, rye, sea water, seafood, shell fish, spinach, well water, wheat, wheat bran, whole grains, fresh unprocessed root vegetables
- Supplements

Research

In post-menopausal women with osteoporosis, women were given supplements of strontium, calcium and vitamin D. There was a 49% risk reduction in the first year and a 41% in the three year period. Strontium ranelate increase bone density during the three years by 14.4% in the lumbar spine and 8.3% at the femoral neck.[651]

Sulfur   (S)
Diallyl disulfide (DADS)
Dimethyl sulfoxide (DMSO)
Methyl Sulfonyl Methane (MSN)

* Nonmetals element.

Possible Uses

* ADD/ADHD, AIDS[652], acne (DMSO)[653], age-related chronic diseases[654], allergies (MSN), Alzheimer's (MSN)[655], amoebic dysentery[656], amyloidosis (DMSO)[657], arteriosclerosis[658], arthritic conditions (MSN)[659], arthritis (DMSO)[660], back/shoulder/wrist pain, bladder infection [661], blood circulation[662], blood pressure control (MSN), blood sugar control[663], bones and teeth health, breast cancer (MSN)[664], burns (DMSO)[665], bursitis (MSN), cancer prevention[666], cardiovascular disease[667], cataract formation[668], cerebral aging[669], cholesterol control[670], chronic fatigue (MSN), chronic pain (MSN), circulatory problems (MSN), colon cancer (DADS)[671], colorectal cancer (garlic)[672], concentration, constipation (MSN), coronary heart disease[673], cramps, Cryptococci meningitis [674], dandruff, diabetes (type 2)[675], digestion, diverticulosis (MSN), dry scalp, dry skin, eczema (MSN), energy, eye inflammation (MSN), fertilizer, food poisoning[676], flu[677], fumigant, fungicide, hair and skin health, hair loss (MSN), head injury (DMSO)[678], headaches, hemorrhoids, hormone-dependent breast cancer (DADS)[679], hormone-independent breast cancer (DADS)[680], inflammation, insomnia, joint inflammation/mobility (MSN)[681], leg cramps (MSN), lower back pain, lupus (MSN), migraines, menopause, mood elevation (MSN), musculoskeletal disorders (MSN)[682], neurological processes, muscle cramps (MSN), obesity

(MSN), oral hygiene (MSN), osteoarthritis (MSN)[683], osteoporosis (MSN), PMS (MSN), periodontal disease (MSN), pneumonia (MSN), prevents paralysis of spinal-cord injury (DMSO)[684], prostate cancer (Allium vegetables)[685], psoriasis, psoriatic arthritis[686], radiation poisoning (MSN), rheumatoid arthritis (MSN), rosacea (MSN)[687], scar tissue (DMSO)[688], scleroderma (DMSO)[689], skin health[690], stomach cancer (garlic)[691], stomach ulcers, stress, stretch marks (MSN), stroke (DMSO)[692], sulfur mustard gas chemical warfare agent[693], sunburn (MSN), tendonitis (MSN), tenosynovitis (MSN), thrombosis formation[694], tuberculosis[695], urinary tract disorders, vaginal yeast infection[696], warts, wound healing (MSN), wrinkles (MSN), yeast infections (MSN)

* Diallyl disulfide (DADS) is an organosulfur compound obtained from garlic, can be diluted to flavor food.
* Dimethyl sulfoxide (DMSO) is an organosulfur synthesized compound from wood pulp, tastes like garlic.
* Methyl Sulfonyl Methane (MSN) is a naturally occurring organic sulfur compound, a metabolite of Dimethyl sulfoxide (DMSO) .

- Other sulfur containing compounds.
  - cysteine
  - diallylsulfide
  - garlic oil extracts
  - lipoid acid
  - N-acetylcysteine
  - mercaptopropionylglycine
  - diallyldisulfide
  - diallyltrisulfide
  - glutathione
  - methionine
  - taurine

Possible Benefits
  - For better absorption, add vitamin C.
  - Disinfects the blood.
  - Resists bacteria.

- Fights allergies.
- Detoxifies the body.
- Protects the cell's protoplasm.
- Aids in oxidation reactions.
- Helps liver produce choline.
- Aids in nutrient absorption.
- Reduces inflammation.
- Manufactures and synthesis for collagen.
- Helps hair and nails grow faster.
- Slows down platelet aggression.
- Stimulates the liver's bile secretions.
- Protects against pollution and harmful radiation emissions.
- Slows down the aging process and extends life.
- Needed for collagen synthesis, prevents dryness and maintains skin elasticity.
- Sulfur amino acids might fight disease.[697]
- Transporter of EDTA into the eye.[698]
- Reduces lactic acid buildup, reduces cramping and sore muscles.
- Protects against radiation and environmental pollution's toxic and harmful effects.
- DMSO crosses the blood-brain barrier.[699]
- DMSO penetrates the skin to get into the bloodstream.[700]
- DMSO Sulfur is a heavy metal detox for aluminum, arsenic, cadmium, lead, mercury and nickel.[701]
- DMSO is an extremely potent free radical scavenger.[702]
- DADS is antimicrobial and insecticidal which attacks insect larva. It also attacks cancer cells but doesn't hurt regular cells.[703]
- DADS has cardiovascular and neuroprotective effects.[704]
- DADS improved glucose tolerance.[705]
- DADS improved renal function.[706]

Properties

- Anti-inflammatory, antibacterial, anticancer, antidiabetic[707], antifungal, antihyperhomocysteinemia[708]antihypertensive[709], antimicrobial, antioxidant[710], antiparasitic, antithrombotic[711], antiviral, cholinesterase properties, cryoprotective, dimethyl sulfoxide (DMSO) is pain reliever, hypercholesterolemic[712], hypolipidemic[713], insecticide, muscle relaxant, radioprotective, transporter

Warnings, Precautions, and Side Effects

- Crush garlic fresh to release allicin, don't cook to maintain healing properties.
- Allergic people can trigger asthma and other allergic reactions, especially when breathing sulfur dioxide.
- Possible allergic reactions are gastrointestinal problems, headache, high fever, hypoglycemia, skin rashes.
- Heating destroys garlic's active allyl sulfur compound which is linked to its anticancer properties.[714]
- Don't confuse sulfa-based drugs (sulfites, sulfates) with the organic sulfur mineral, the drugs can cause allergic reactions to a person who is fine with organic sulfur foods. Be prudent when using sulfur based foods and check for toxicity.

Food Sources

- Asparagus, Brussels sprouts, cabbage, cauliflower, cayenne, dairy products, dried beans, eggs, fish, *garlic, horseradish, horsetail (herb), kale, land cress, legumes, meats, nettle, onions, organ meats, parsley, poultry, soybeans, turnips, watercress, wheat germ
- Amino acids: L-cysteine, L-cystine, L-lysine, and L-methionine
- Alpha-lipoid acid

Research

Garlic has over 20 kinds of sulfide compounds coming from a few different sulfur-containing amino acids. Their functions are distinctive, differing one from one another.[715]

Vanadium (V)
Vanadyl sulfate   Vanadate

- Transitional metals element.
- It is assumed to be possibly an essential trace mineral.[716]
- A deficiency hasn't been identified.[717]

Possible Uses

- Anemia, blood pressure control, blood sugar control, body builders, bone health, breast cancer[718], cancer prevention, cardiovascular disease[719], cholesterol control, coronary artery disease[720], diabetes[721], Ehrlich ascites carcinoma[722], gastrointestinal problems, heart disease, human B cell lymphoma[723], hyperlipemia[724], hypertension[725], hypoglycemia, ischemic/reperfusion-induced heart injury[726], kidney cancer[727], larynx carcinoma[728], lung cancer[729], nasopharyngeal carcinoma[730], ovary carcinoma[731], prostate cancer[732], runny nose, sore throat, syphilis[733], T-cell leukemia[734], Lewis lung carcinoma[735], testicular cancer[736], triglyceride control, tuberculosis[737], water retention, weight training, wheezing

Possible Benefits
- Works in concert with molybdenum.
- Red blood cell production.
- Vital for cellular metabolism.
- Needed for tooth and bone formation.
- Role in reproduction and growth.
- Inhibits cholesterol synthesis.
- Stored in bones, kidney, and liver.
- Might work like insulin.[738]
- Has insulin-like actions.[739]
- Dietary vanadyl sulfate has chemo protective properties.[740]

- Vanadyl metformin (diabetes) is made from a Vanadium compound.

Possible Deficiency
- Impaired reproductive ability.
- Increased infant mortality.

Properties
- Anticancer[741], antineoplastic[742], antioxidant, antiproliferative[743], chemo protective[744], cytostatic[745], metal antitumor agent[746], photogenic[747], proliferative[748]

Warnings, Precautions, and Side Effects
- Use in moderation, can be toxic in high doses.
- Dust might irritate the eyes and upper respiratory system: chest pain, conjunctivitis, cough, nasal hemorrhage, rhinitis, sore throat and wheezing.[749]
- Tobacco decreases uptake.
- Interaction between vanadium (antagonist) and chromium, so take at different times.
- Do not take in high doses, toxic symptoms might include: abdominal pain, anorexia, cramps, depression, dehydration, diarrhea, fatigue, gas, lesions to kidney or spleen[750], nausea, nose bleeds, pulmonary hemorrhage[751], purple green or green tongue, renal tubular necrosis[752], stomach pain, uric acid increased[753], vomiting, weight loss or death.[754]
- Drug interactions with MAO inhibitors, phenothiazine's, ethylenediaminetetracetic acid.
- Anticoagulant or antiplatelet drug bleeding interactions may occur with aspirin, clopidogrel (Plavix), heparin, and warfarin (Coumadin).[755]

Food Sources

- Black pepper, cabbage, carrots, chicken white meat, corn, dill, egg yolk fish, gelatin, grains, green beans, leafy green vegetables, meat, mushroom, oats, olive oil, olives, parsley, peanut butter, radishes, sea food, sea weed, seeds, skim milk, snap beans, soybeans, vegetable oils, whole grains

Research

Vanadium compounds exercise protective effects in opposition to chemical carcinogenesis. Its anti-tumor properties inhibit cellular tyrosine phosphates and phosphorylases, the two leading factors in apoptosis or tumor suppression. Further, it reduces cell-cycle arrest, cytotoxic properties through DNA cleavage. It might inhibit cancer cell metastatic possibilities and overturn antineoplastic drug resistance. Vanadium also has low toxicity, is well tolerated, and is a valuable non-platinum, metal antitumor agent.[756]

Zinc   (Zn)
Zinc chloride   Zinc citrate   Zinc gluconate

- Transitional metals element.
- Essential trace element in which the immune system depends upon it.

Possible Uses

- Acne[757], acrodermatitis enteropathica[758], acute diarrhea[759], acute ethanol-induced liver damage[760], age-related macular degeneration[761], alcoholics[762], alcoholic cirrhosis[763], Alzheimer's[764], anorexia[765], appetite loss, atherosclerosis[766], auto-immune diseases[767], brain development[768], brain function[769], bulimia[770], bulimirexic, cadmium (zinc pretreatment)[771], cancer, childhood mental and physical growth and development[772], childhood infectious diseases[773], childhood respiratory illnesses[774], chronic fatigue, chronic hepatitis C[775], chronic pancreatitis[776], cold sores, colds[777], coronary heart disease[778], critically ill[779], dermatitis, dental plaque[780], diabetes, diarrhea childhood morbidity[781], eating disorders[782], eczema, elderly infection[783], gum health, hair loss, immune system, infantile protein-energy malnutrition[784], influenza (H1N1, H2N2, H3N2)[785], lactation, leishmaniosis[786], leprosy[787], lethargy, liver disease[788], malnutrition, neurological disorders[789], night blindness[790], obesity, pale skin, pancreatic cystic fibrosis[791], retinal mobilization[792], several malignancies[793], shigellosis[794], sickle cell disease infection[795], skin conditions, sperm motility, stress, thought clarity, tinnitus, vision loss, WWI substitute penicillin treatment, white spots under finger nails, Wilson's disease[796], wounds

Possible Benefits
- Essential for cell proliferation and differentiation.
- Essential for the immune system.
- Needed for DNA synthesis and mitosis.
- Helps the body absorb vitamin antioxidants.
- Necessary to make protein, helps to string long chain amino acids together.
- Part of the hormone insulin, aids in transporting vitamin A to where it can be used.
- Aids bone metabolism along with calcium.
- Increases natural killer cell activity.
- Essential for the thymic hormones.
- Helps white blood cells.
- Responsible for T-cells development.
- Aids with cell-mediated immune functions.[797]
- Fights oxidative stress.[798]
- Zinc and copper are essential in stimulating the pituitary thus signaling the thyroid to create more thyroid hormones.
- Zinc and copper also aids in collagen formation, slows down bone deterioration.
- Teams up with vitamin A to protect skin cells.
- Affects the release of stored vitamin A in the liver.
- Aids vitamin E in the blood.
- Slows *N*-methyl-*N*-nitrosourea and testosterone-induced prostatic preneoplastic development.[799]
- Simple and cheap way for elderly people and hemodialysis patients with infection to increase the immune system.[800]
- Offers hope for genital herpes, topical zinc and L-lysine helped it not multiply, although not a cure.[801]

Possible Deficiency
- Phytates block absorption.[802]
- Loss of immunity defenses.[803]

- Growth stunted, hypogonadism, immune system dysfunction.[804]
- Alcoholics, elderly and hospitalized people are more susceptible to bacterial sepsis mortality because of zinc deficiency.[805]
- Causes fast deterioration of the thymus along with T-cell helper function loss.[806]
- Might increase the risk of cancer.[807]

Possible Detriment
- Too much zinc might cause prostate cancer.[808]

Properties
- Anti-inflammatory, antibacterial, anticancer, antioxidant, antiviral, bactericide

Warnings, Precautions, and Side Effects
- Wilson disease (copper build-up).
- Do not use if pregnant or breastfeeding, or give to small infants. Consult physician.
- Whole grain breads may have phytates that binds the zinc and other minerals from absorption, yeast counteracts the phytates, unleavened bread has the phytates intact.
- Too much can depress the immune system, cause anemia, skin outbreaks, increase blood cholesterol, and symptoms like scurvy.
- Doses of 100 milligrams of zinc daily can depress the immune system while does under can enhance it.
- High doses can cause effects like a zinc deficiency.
- Men who took less than 100 mg/day supplements in zinc had lower risk of prostate cancer than men who took more than 100 mg/day of zinc.[809]
- Cirrhosis of liver, diabetes, diarrhea, kidney disease and fiber can lower zinc levels.

- The proper zinc/copper balance needs to be maintained, hard water can disturb that balance.

Food Sources
- Beef liver, black-eyed peas, Brazil nuts, brewer's yeast, buckwheat, *calves liver, cashews, cheddar cheese, chickpeas, *chicken heart, chicken liver, clams, crab, eggs, fish, ground beef, herring, lamb, legumes, lentils, lima beans, liver, meats, mushrooms, mussels, oatmeal, *oysters, peanuts, pecans, poultry, pumpkin seeds, sardines, seafood, seeds, sesame seeds, soy lecithin, soybeans, sunflower seeds, Swiss cheese, tourla, tuna, turkey, wheat germ, whole grains

*** Best of the Rest**

Research
Another method to stop the development of retroviruses, along with HIV, is to aim the zinc ions ejection from significant zinc finger viral proteins.[810]

Recipes

Zinc Folk Remedy for sore throat or cold
- On first inkling of cold or sore throat
- Eat something light first, zinc can cause stomach upset on empty stomach
- Suck on 30-50 mg zinc tablet until dissolved (yes, yucky)
- Lozenges at 12.5 mg for children
- Do not drink anything
- Repeat in 12-24 hours
- Should kill infection

Dr. Chase's Recipes 1902   Eye Inflammation[811]
> • If sore eyes shed much water, put a little of the oxide of zinc into a vial of water and use it rather freely--it will soon cure that difficulty.

Zinc Dental Plaque Mouth Wash
- 7/8 of a quart of water
- 1/8 quart of vodka
- 2 T. Xylitol sugar
- Optional: 2 T. hydrogen peroxide
- Colloidal zinc
- Add favorite flavorings, according to taste:
  - Cinnamon, citrus, mint, spearmint, wintergreen
- Swish and spit

GEOPHAGIA

The practice of eating clay, chalk or dirt has been considered by Western medical practitioners as abnormal behavior, and labeled those who practiced this behavior as having a DSM IV psychological disorder, called pica.

Eating clay is a practice demonstrated world-wide, by humans, as well as many animals. Historically, clay was eaten as treatments for bacterial infections, cholera, poison and the plague.

Today, pregnant women are eating clay and soil. In some cases, scientists are finding the clay to be rich in minerals, such as calcium and iron, which are beneficial to the woman, as well as the fetus. People are also using clay for increasing trace minerals, digestive problems, detoxification, chronic infections, heavy metal poisoning and so much more.

TRACE MINERALS

"Sick Soils, Sick Plants, Sick People." [812]
--by Spice Williams-Crosby

Approximately 95% of the human body's mass is made up of the elements: calcium, carbon, hydrogen, oxygen, phosphorus, chlorine, magnesium, potassium, sodium and sulfur and the rest are trace minerals. Even though it looks like the trace minerals are not very important, they are. As we have learned from some of the above minerals, each has a purpose, a job to do in helping us to remain healthy and if we are deficient, then our body is balance is off and we can suffer dire consequences.

Even when I was a child, and that was a long time ago, I heard how we were depleting our soil of vital nutrients. So, do you think it's any better nowadays?

It isn't.

About 50% of our modern commercially-grown foods receives their mineral content from fertilizers because the soil is depleted of these vital nutrients. Humans need approximately 60 trace minerals. Andy yet what we see from these fertilizers, the plants receive six macronutrients of calcium, magnesium, nitrogen, phosphorus, potassium and sulfur and eight micronutrients like boron, chlorine, copper, iron , manganese, molybdenum, nickel and zinc. Therefore, even though the fertilizers are adding minerals to the soil, it's not enough. Our food supply is lacking the vital macro and micro ionic trace minerals.

And then when we examine our food sources even further, we notice our food has been genetically modified organisms (GMOs). Only heaven and Monsanto knows how the how DNA has been changed, surely, the average person has no clue. And then, our food is drenched in pesticide poison, is it any wonder why so many Americans are getting sick?

Actually, most people probably don't think about trace minerals…don't care. We don't see how it is needed or even whether it applies to us. After all, trace minerals are just tiny things that are rarely talked about.

Does it matter whether we know about minerals or not?

Are you tired of being sick yet?

If you are… then understand, our food sucks up minerals from the earth, then we eat the foods. If that earth is poor quality, the foods we eat are poor quality. Sure, it may fill our gut, but our body isn't receiving the nourishment it needs to operate at maximum performance, heck, not even minimum performance levels in many cases.

Look around us at the people who are aging, they're falling apart. Nowadays, we just accept it as the norm, but it shouldn't be. It should show us, something is wrong. Food addictions, our bellies are fatter, we eat more, yet we don't feel better. Why?

Why are people falling apart?

It's not just the elderly people's problem but our children are becoming obese and developing type 2 diabetes, and was once considered an old person's disease.

I think we're slowly starving to death even though our bellies are fat. I believe we're craving food because our bodies are missing something it needs but we don't know what, so they continue to eat, hoping to feel better.

In the meantime, people are dying slowly and painfully. Their body ridden with disease and deteriorating because they aren't getting the vital nutrition their body craves. I think our food is poisoning us, white sugar, white bread, bleached, then enriched with less nutrients than the original food. The foods we love are fattening, yet void of nutrition.

Health care costs are skyrocketing. Medicare benefits are being cut. Isn't it time to wake up? Isn't it time for us to learn how to eat right and take care of ourselves, in order to live a better quality of life?

And so, what do we do?

Unfortunately, we don't change we diet.

Instead, we run to the doctor for help. Modern medicine has the answer. And the doctor gives them a new little pill. Creating health?

Are we crazy?

If we keep following this path we are.

The problem is, you might be next, if you don't change now.

**"There is nothing magical about trace elements--
they are simply essential."**
--Mette M. Berger, MD, PhD[813]

So, where can we find trace minerals?
- Daily supplements
- Colloidal mineral solutions
- Mineral water
- Hard water
- Ionic minerals
- Organic clay and shaljit
- Fulvic and humic acid
- Mineral salts
- Blackstrap molasses
- Peat, mumie, coal-derived HA
    - Sphagnum peat
- Organically grown foods, particularly root vegetables.
- Organic grass-fed organ meats: brain, heart, liver along with vitamin A, D, and long-chain fatty acids (omega 3

WATER

Water is a necessity for life. Nothing lives without it. It's the most important source of energy. It generates the power to energize every body cell, electrically and magnetically.

Every cell in our body needs water. That's because we are mostly water.
- Blood is approximately 94% water.
- Brain is approximately 85% water.
- Lungs are approximately 90% water.
- Blood is approximately 83% water.
- All other tissues are approximately 75% water.

Possible Uses
- Acid-alkaline imbalance, aging, anxiety, constipation, dehydration, depression, digestion problems, excessive fatigue, gastritis, glaucoma, heart health, high blood pressure, joint lubricant, kidney detox, liver detox, muscle strength, nutrient assimilation, skin hydration, stress, weight management, wrinkled skin

F. Batmanghelidj, M.D., an Iranian physician makes a persuasive argument that continual dehydration is the cause for numerous serious health problems like: angina; arthritis; asthma; autoimmune diseases; back pain; blood pressure; cholesterol; colitis; diabetes; fibromyalgia; heartburn; lower back pain; migraines; and rheumatoid joint pain[814]. He believes that many of our sickness are because we're really thirsty. We're not getting enough water. He thinks we should drink sufficient water, not just resort to medications.

Possible Benefits
- Needed for absorption, circulation, digestion, and excretion.
- Breaks down foods, vitamins and minerals.
- Foundation of blood and blood glucose.
- Foundation of lymph system.
- Lubricates organs.

- Lubricates mucus which protects lining and membranes in stomach and respiratory system.
- Body temperature regulation.
- Increases enzyme production.
- Protects from DNA damage.
- Supports the immune system's effectiveness.
- Normalizes blood-manufacturing in the bone marrow.
- Without water, food eaten receives no energy value at all.
- Boosts red blood cell oxygen effectiveness in the lungs.
- Reverses alcohol, caffeine and other addictive drug urges.[815]

Maintaining Hydration Creates Good Health
- Drink 1-2 glasses plain water first thing in the morning.
    - Don't use flavored drinks as substitutes for water, it becomes food and changes the molecular structure, it has to be…just plain old water.
- Wait about 1/2 hour before eating food.
    - Water enters stomach and, activates the glands into releasing chemical (hormone) to cover the stomach lining and protect it from the release of hydrochloric acid that happens when we eat food.
- Water and chemical (hormone) enters the small intestine where the chemical stays awaiting the food.
- The free water leaves the small intestine and goes to all of the body's cells, hydrating them.
- Residual water is driven back into the stomach to water (hydrolyze) the food.
- Our energy doesn't actually come from our food.
- Our energy comes from the water that deposits the hydrogen atom in food.
- Food gives the vitamins and minerals to stay healthy.

Not Maintaining Hydration Creates Bad Health

If you don't drink 1-2 glasses plain water before eating food, then didn't wait 20-30 minutes, your body:
- Borrows water from itself, thus compromising another tissue or organ.
- When the body borrows water from:
  - The blood, the arteries constrict, forcing the heart to pump harder in order to move the thicker blood, or "high blood pressure."
  - The brain, it results in a dull headache, maybe a migraine.
  - The colon or small intestine, an abnormal function causes constipation.
  - The lungs, causes shortness of breath, leads to asthma and other breathing problems.
  - The lungs and heart, may lead to angina pain, and possibly to a heart attack.
  - The muscles, you may cause shortness of breath, get an asthma attack, get angina pain or leg cramps.

How Much Water Do I Need?
- 1/2 body weight in ounces per day.
- Space intake throughout day.
- 1/2 hour before and 1/2 hour after eating, drink again.
- Drink anytime, especially when you're thirsty, but before you get thirsty preferably.
- The higher the elevation, the more water is needed.

Dehydration
- Body loses 1/2-1 gallon water daily.
- Dehydration prevents sex hormone production, causing impotence.
- Causes toxic deposits in issue, organs, and the skin.

Causes of Dehydration
- Burns, diarrhea, diabetes, not drinking water, sweating, vomiting.

Symptoms of Dehydration

- Thirst, dry mouth
- Weakness, muscle cramps
- Lethargy
- Nausea, vomiting
- Heart palpitations
- Lightheaded or dizzy when standing
- Confusion, decreased mental capacity
- Dull headache
- Not hungry
- Dark colored urine
    - Healthy urine is uncolored to light yellow colored.
- Infant soft spot on head is sunken, no armpit/groin sweat.
- Poor sleep pattern

Preventing Water Loss

- Obtain water before dehydrated.
- Get electrolytes.
- Take it easy.
- Stay cool.
- Seek shelter.
- Avoid fatty foods.
- Eat fruit and vegetables for water.
- Stay in shaded or covered area.
- Avoid caffeinated drinks, they're a diuretic.
- Avoid alcohol, also a diuretic which takes water out of the body.
- Avoid sugary drinks, sports drinks without sugar and artificial colors.

Warning, Precautions and Side Effects

- Some cities put chlorine as well as ammonia (choramine) to disinfect their water.

Research

Dyspepic pain can be relieved by drinking water.[816]

In a water drinking test, the patients with visual field progression (glaucoma) progressed significantly after drinking water.[817]

Calcium absorption from calcium rich mineral water is accessible for intestinal absorption and is suggested for older people and those who are lactose intolerant.[818]

Consumption of a high calcium mineral water in postmenopausal women with low calcium intake can repair a calcium deficiency and reduce age-related bone loss.[819]

Sodium rich carbonated water can reduce the risk of cardiovascular disease and the metabolic syndrome in postmenopausal women.[820]

Whenever I talk about water throughout this book, I'm not talking about tap (contaminated) water. I'm encouraging the use of non-contaminated water. This can come in a variety of forms, like filtered water, bottled water, mineral water, hard water, spring water or well water. If these aren't available, boil your water and filter it. Seek the best water you can for your personal use.

Electrolytes

- Electrolytes are ion salts, essential for humans.
- They are positively or negatively charged signature.
- Found in a solution, conducts electricity, and is electrolyzed by it.
- Contains free ions.
- Without electrolytes, the body can't communicate within itself.
- Each mineral is an acid, base or salt. The human body can't move without these essential minerals for they are connected to the electrical impulses that activate our total nervous system.

Colloidal vs. Ionic Minerals

- Minerals are found in two forms: Colloidal and Ionic.

Colloidal Minerals
- Minerals in high concentrations are evenly suspended in a stable liquid form.
- Because of their large size and not having an electrical charge, they are not easily absorbed by the body.
- Swish in mouth to enhance absorption.
- Strong metallic taste.
- Not easily absorbed because they aren't electrically charged.
- Unable to cross digestive tract cell membranes.
- The amount of assimilation depends on the size (atomic is best) and absorbency of the mineral. The larger the size, the less absorbability therefore the lesser the value the mineral has for health benefits. Most colloidal minerals are too large.
- High colloidal ratio products say "Staying Power."

Ionic Minerals

- Ionic minerals have an intrinsic positive or negative charge.
- Natural occurring from plants
- Swish in mouth to enhance absorption.
- Bio-available immediately.
- Topically effective and fast acting.
- Less sediment and light sensitivity.
- Have a nutritional value.
- Electrical impulses are important to digestion, heart, muscles, and nerves.
- They may have too many or too few electrons, making them unstable.
- This makes it possible to bond with water so the body can absorb it easier, since we are made up mostly of water, it makes for easier absorption.
- Negatively or positively charged electrical signatures unite to create billions of tiny chemical or electrical processes to facilitate nutrient movement, transportation across cell membranes and through the intestinal wall, directing body functions, like muscle contractions, nerve transmissions, regulating amino acids, enzymes and hormones.
- When mineral atoms link with oppositely charged atoms, they share electrons, forming different mineral complexes along with stability, like sodium chloride and potassium chloride, wherein the chloride being negatively charged ion and the sodium and potassium being positively charged.

Positive Charged Ions	**Negative Charged Ions**
Aluminum	Nitride
Hydrogen	Hydride
Sodium	Chloride
Chlorate	Nitrate

Calcium

Potassium

Magnesium

Phosphorous

Lithium

Silver

Barium

Zinc

Bismuth

Phosphate

Cesium

Strontium

Iron

Copper

Cobalt

Carbonate (bicarbonate)

Tin

Bromate

Lead

Mercury

Rubidium

Hydrogen sulfate

Hydroxide

Bicarbonate

Phosphate

Fluoride

Iodide

Oxide

Sulfide

Phosphide

Sulfate

Bromide

Arsenide

Cyanide

Carbonate

Hydrogen

Amide

Bromite

Iodate

Iodite

Peroxide

Thiosulfate

Borate

Oxalate

Oxide

Thiocyanate

One mineral, positive or negative, without the other creates an imbalanced distribution of electrons. This can cause acute and chronic diseases. The object is to create balance.

There are laboratory tests to check for imbalances in each different mineral. For more information, please see article, "Electrolytes" updated by David C. Dugdale, III, MD (http://www.nlm.nih.gov/medlineplus/ency/article/002350.htm)

"No Cellular functions can be produced correctly
if the body isn't receiving all the minerals and trace
elements the metabolism needs....
It so happens that all degenerative diseases originate,
to one degree or another, in a severe mineral
depletion of the body."[821]
--Dr. Robert LaFave,
US Metabolic Research Center

Fulvic Acid (FA)   Humic Acid (HA)
Oxifulvic Acid

- Edible dirt for human consumption.
- Powerful natural organic electrolyte.
- Water soluble in all different pH waters.
- FA is water-soluble and has all pH conditions. It is acidic, alkaline and neutral.
- Derived from prehistoric plant material along with fulvic shale but also derived from decaying plant matter.
- Organic material, made up of beneficial microbes, occurs naturally in plants and soil, and resides in small amounts in clay.
- Folvates are the salts from fulvic ionic minerals (fulvic acid) which is an organic electrolyte coming from clay.
- 60-70+ Macro and Micro trace minerals in ionic (nano) form.
- Low molecular-weight aids in 100% cell permeability.
- Can carry over 60 times its weight in vitamins and minerals and aid absorption into cells.
- Powerful natural herbomineral electrolyte, carrier molecule for deep tissue and toxin removal.
- Ultramicroscopic substance with unique messaging system comes from the decomposition of organic material and activates with contact from a living organism.

• Most research has been done for creating healthy plants but now, the eye has turned to seeing how it can benefit humans.

• FA is more abundantly found in water, approximately 9-10 times higher than HA.[822]

• HA is richly found in soil and along streams, it is found to be 50% of the broken up organic carbon material where FA is 90-95%.[823]

• HA was formed from dead plant matter and is found in coal, dystrophic lakes, humus, ocean water and peat.

• Can come in salts, esters or derivatives and used in cream, gel, ointment, paste, or powder or solution.

Possible Uses

• Abrasions, acne[824], alkalinizes body, allergic reactions[825], Alzheimer's[826], anemia[827], angina, animal feed/health (peat)[828], anxiety, arteriosclerosis[829], arthritis[830], asthma[831], athlete's foot[832], autism, bacterial ear infection[833], bed sores[834], bipolar, bladder, bleeding, blood clots, blood pressure control, blood sugar stabilizer[835], body odor[836], bone regeneration (mumie)[837], brain functioning, bronchitis, Brukitt's lymphoma[838], burns, cancer[839], candida albicans[840], cervical cancer[841], chronic fatigue, cognitive stimulation[842], colds, cow's mastitis, cuts[843], diabetes[844], diabetic gangrene[845], digestion, digestive tract ulcers, eczema[846], emotional stress, energy[847], epidemic hemorrhagic fever[848], esophagus cancer[849], eye diseases - bacterial/ fungal/ viral[850], fever, fibromyalgia[851], gastric problems[852], gastroenterological bleeding[853], Graves disease[854], HIV[855], heavy metal soil detoxification[856], hemorrhaging[857], Herpes simplex virus-1[858], herpes zoster[859], Human Papilloma virus[860], hyperacidity[861], hypercholesterolemia[862], hypertension[863], inflammation[864], insomnia[865], influenza (H1N1, H3N2,H5N1)[866], intestinal problems, Kaposi sarcoma herpes virus[867], kidney, lead chelation[868], leprosy[869], liver, lupus[870], lung infection[871], mastitis (cattle), mental clarity, migraines[872], mineral retention, multiple sclerosis[873], muscle performance[874], nervous disorders, nutrient absorption[875], osteoporosis (mumie)[876], parasites, poison ivy, poison oak, pollutant detoxification, poxviruses (Secomet V)[877], psoriasis, radiation detoxification, rashes, reduces need for antibiotics, rheumatoid arthritis[878],SARS (Secomet V)[879], scarring, soil decontamination, spider bites, stamina[880], stress management, surgical shock, surgical stitches[881], thrombosis[882], thyroid hormones, toxins, thyroid tumors[883], toxin elimination[884], tuberculosis, ulcerous colon infection[885], ulcerous cornea infection[886], urinary tract, vasculitis[887], Von Willebrand disease[888], weakness, weight loss, wounds[889]

• Most of these are alternative medicine, traditional or folk remedies use and I didn't find any research to back them. It appears that FA can not be synthesized by scientists and duplicated by pharmaceutical companies, therefore, no drugs.

Possible Benefits of Fulvic Acid
• Water-soluble and fat-soluble organic electrolyte.
• Oral chelation, binding metals to organic materials.
• Metabolic detoxification.
• Increases thymus gland size, age decreases it.
• It is able to conduct electrical current, balances electrical cell potential and maintains the electrical potential of the cell.
• Energy-rich, bio-electric charged transporter.
• Absorb positive and negative electrical charges neutralizing free radicals.

- Stimulates metabolism and immune system response.
- Alkalinizes the body extremely quick.
- Stimulates blood circulation and coagulation.
- Fulvic acid and humic acid act as one to eliminate unwanted salt acids that harden cell wells, thus producing essential cell permeability.
- Increases macrophages and killer T-cells production.
- Encourages granulocytes and cytokines manufacturing, including interferon-alpha, interferon-beta, interferon-gamma, and tumor necrosis factor-alpha.[890]
- Improves the availability of nutrients, makes trace minerals and trace metals more accessible to the organism, not metallic minerals.
- Close involvement with enzymes[891], especially respiratory catalysts.
- Increases alkaline phosphates, invertase, and transaminase enzyme activity.
- Dissolves silica to release mineral nutrients.
- Magnifies vitamins and herbs, breaking them down into the simplest ionic form.
- Fulvic acid (ionic form) makes iron available to bone marrow.
- Increases and restores blood circulation and carries oxygen in the blood.
- HA activates T-lymphocytes.[892]
- HA inactivates heavy metals, hydro-carbons, pesticides, petroleum products, polyaromatic radioactive metals and toxins.[893]
- Stimulates cytokine production (interferon-alpha, interferon-beta, interferon-gamma, tumor necrosis factor-alpha) which means humic extracts can search for, discriminate and kills cancer cells.[894]
- FA doesn't show to definitely destroy cancer cells, but works in the immune system as a regulating agent and is often used in combination with anti-cancer medicines.[895]

- FA activated and stimulated white blood cells, encouraging healing, turning inorganic calcium into organic and into a bio-active cellular regenerative bone growth, also stimulating cellular growth and regeneration, and inhibiting HIV.[896]
- FA has antiviral activity and contains Secomet V which has been found to fight against SARS and the poxviruses.[897]
- Stimulates white blood cells, encourages healing.[898]
- Changes inorganic calcium into organic calcium which aids in bio-active cellular regenerative bone growth.[899]
- Stimulates cellular growth and regeneration, inhibiting HIV.[900]
- Strong humoral immune stimulation.[901]
- Can be made into a ointment, paste, powder or solution.[902]

Properties of Fulvic Acid

- Analgesic, anti-aging, anti-anxiety, anti-inflammatory[903],anti-influenza, anti-lipid-peroxidative activity, antibacterial[904], anticancer, antidiabetic, antifungal[905], antimicrobial, antioxidant, antimutagenic[906], antipathogens[907], antitoxic[908], antitumor[909], antiviral[910], apoptotic[911], coagulant[912], heavy metal chelator[913], immunodulatory[914], nootropic, ovogenic, photo-protective[915], powerful electrolyte, powerful free radical scavenger, spermatogenic, vermifuge

Warning, Precautions and Side Effects

- Too much may cause diarrhea or constipation.
- **Chlorine reacts negatively with fulvic acid**, causing deadly carcinogenic production (THMs and MX). Chlorine is the poisonous perpetrator, not the humic acid.[916]

• One 1000 mg. vitamin C or ascorbic acid will remove the chlorine from water in a bathtub or there is the Sonaki Vitamin C shower head, or there are chlorine filters that might remove the chlorine although maybe not the chloramine.

Research

Even though scientists across the world have published many thousands of research papers about the effects of "Fulvic acid"on living matter, public exposure has been restricted due to the inability to commercialize this substance.[917]

"Transfer factor," a scientific term, is "a substance that is produced and secreted by lymphocyte which has not been sensitized confers on it the same immunological specificity as the sensitized cell." Fulvic acid appears to have an incredible amount of commonalities with the transfer factor, too much for it to be considered accidental. And because fulvic acid's production cycles engages in such a varied spectrum of living organisms, this might explain its remarkable immune stimulating powers that go beyond the transfer factor.[918]

Within a hospital's care, studies demonstrate that patients with incurable epidemic Hemorrhagic Fever treated with humic extracts showed circulation restoration, clot removal, and bleeding to stop. It was also discovered that humic extract was anti-viral which bolstered and regulated the immune system significantly.[919]

Recipe

Fulvic & Humic Acid Bath
- Up to 10% fulvic/humic extract water solution.
- Extender saturation can be successful for internal and external conditions.
- Said to cure the flu and common cold.
- 92% rate success for treating skin ulcers.[920]
- Clinical baths treat serious disease like autoimmune disorders with bone, joint, muscle and tendon disorders, along with severe rheumatoid arthritis[921], viral diseases and enhancing the immune system.[922]

Shilajit   Shilajit Ramayana

• Oozing blackish-brown mineral pitch seeping from between rock layers in the Himalayans and Hindukush mountain range.

• Used in ancient times as well as Hindu Ayurvedic medicine today.

• The active ingredient with the most healing properties is fulvic acid.

• Contains approximately 84 minerals, including copper, iron, lead, silver, zinc and trace minerals. Main active constituent is fulvic acid.

4 Varieties

  • Lauha shilajit is common in the Himalayas and is considered to have the most effective therapeutic benefits.
  • Rajat is silver shilajit and the color is white.
  • Savrana Shilajit is gold and the color is red.
  • Tamra is copper and is blue in color.

• The Indian Shilajit Ayurveda/Siddha traditional Hindu medicine lacks substantial evidence to verify it's abilities.[923]

Traditional Hindu Uses

  • Abdomen enlargement, aging, allergies, Alzheimer's[924], anxiety[925], bladder stones[926], blood sugar control, body pain[927], cardiac, chronic fatigue syndrome[928], chronic fever[929], cognitive stimulation[930], constipation, cough, dementia[931], depression[932], diabetes, diarrhea, digestion, dysuria[933], epilepsy[934], eye disorders [935], general tonic, hemorrhoids, high altitude cerebral edema[936], hypertension[937], hypoxia (high altitude problems)[938],

immune system, insanity, insomnia[939], jaundice[940], lack of appetite, lethargy[941], microbial gastro-intestinal infection[942], malignant tumor[943], muscular degradation, nervous system,
nausea, parasites[944], phthisis (body wasting)[945], pulmonary edema[946], radiation protection (high intensity UV)[947], rectal distula[948], rejuvenator, scrofula[949], skin problems[950], stress, tiredness, thyroid disorders[951], tuberculous cervical lymphadenitis[952], worms, vomiting

Possible Benefits
- Used with milk makes it a strong supplement for fighting weakness.
- Potential for modulating orofacial pain.[953]
- Shilajit improves CoQ10's mitochondrial benefits and sustains active
ubiquinol form levels.[954]

Properties of Shalajit
- Adaptogenic[955], anodyne[956], anti-AIDS[957], anti-aging, anti-anxiety[958], anti-allergic, anti-lipid peroxidative activity[959], anti-asthmatic[960], anti-inflammatory, anti-ulcer[961], antibacterial, antidiabetic, antifungal, antioxidant[962], antiretroviral[963], antiseptic, antiviral[964], cytotoxic[965], immunodulatory,[966] immunostimulant[967], laxative, nootropic (enhances learning, memory)[968]

Constituents
- Living matter, bio-active on cellular level.

- 60-80% humus organic matter (smells like cow urine), non-humic organic metabolites, alkanol esters, amino acids, fulvic acid, mostly humic acid, calcium benzoate, benzoic acid, hippuric acid, uronic acids, phenolic glucosides, several phenolic, fatty acid, microbial metabolites, organic plant material, albuminoids, vegetable matter, dibenzo-alphapyrones, amino acid peptides, nucleic acids, polysaccharides, muco-polysaccharides.
- RNA and DNA from organic plant photosynthetic material remain intact creating ultimately an intense intricate organic carbonaceous material.

Smectite - Kaolinite Clay Groups

- Originates from volcanic ash.
- Contains fulvic acid.
- Mineral clays might have trace minerals.
- Highly alkaline.
- Some are negative charged, some not.
- Colloidal electrolytes.[969]

Sodium Bentonite (montmorillonite)
  - Strong sodium chloride concentration.[970]
  - Swelling and ionization.

In this book, I will focus primarily on Calcium Bentonite Clay for health benefits.

Calcium Bentonite Clay
(montmorillonite, non-swelling)
Pascalite Clay   Carmargo Earth

- Originates from volcanic ash.
- Contains fulvic acid.
- Highly alkaline.
- Negative charge.

Possible Benefits

- Abrasions[971], acne, addiction dependency, aflatoxin-induced disease[972], anemia, animal feed supplements, arthritis, avian flu (H5N1)[973], avulsions[974], bone formation, bowel regulation, brown recluse spider bite, burns[975], calluses, cataracts, chemical leaching, chicken pox irritation and itching, colitis, colon cleanse, cuts, degenerative diseases, deodorant, detoxifier, diaper rash, diarrhea[976], dietary mineral supplement, digestive aid, draws out impurities, drinking water defluoridation[977], eczema, environmental contamination, excessive bleeding[978], explosion-burn victim, facial masks, fibromyalgia, fiddle back spider bites, gangrene, gastrointestinal protectors[979], germicidal, HIV-1[980], heavy metal removal[981], hemorrhoids, hypoglycemia, immune system, influenza (H3N2)[982], insect bites[983], intestinal distress, intestinal problems, irritable bowel syndrome (IBS)[984], joint disease, lacerations[985], lead chelation[986], neuropathic, oil production, organ health, osteoarthritis, osteoporosis[987], pain, peptic ulcers[988], poisons, pollutants, radiation decontamination (cesium, cobalt, strontium)[989], rheumatic inflammation[990], skin care, psoriasis, pyorrhea, skin problems, toothpaste, toxins, ulcers[991], wounds[992], open wounds
- Used to decontaminate water against dysentery or radiation.

- See Calcium for more information.

Possible Benefits
- Powerful healing clay (internal and external).
- Bentonite clay is composed of montmorillonite.
- Montmorillonite clay has some fulvic acid.[993]
- Trace minerals for mineral deficiencies.
- Absorbs contaminants, impurities, heavy metals, toxins.
- Flexible crystal lattice-like atomic structure.
- Negative electrical charge on platelet nano particles.
- Collects minerals through electro kinetics like a magnet and sponge.
- Nano delivery system for anticancer drugs.[994]
- Deposits calcium into bone matrix.
- Shelf-life is indefinite.

Possible Properties
- Anesthetic, antibacterial, antidiuretic[995], antifungal, antihistaminic, antihypertensive, antimicrobial, antitoxin, antitumor, antiulcerative, antiviral[996]
- Smecties is a major bentonite component.

Constituents
- Pascalite clay contains approximately 67 minerals: aluminum, calcium, copper, gold,iron, magnesium, silicon, silver, sodium, titanium, trace minerals along with protein and enzymes.

Warning, Precautions, and Side Effects
- If using clay, use in moderation.
- Can cause constipation.
- Do not inhale.
- Some people have great concerns about eating clay and believe it's detrimental to one's health.

Research

A chemical engineer, Harvey C. Lisle, a biodynamic specialist, recognized Pascalite rock dust is "alive," and radiates energy about 100 feet and has the power to counteract toxic energy. If one places it above or below a microwave or TV set, tests demonstrate harmful electric energies are eliminated. It also rejuvenates "dead" soil.[997]

Montmorillonite didn't have a bactericidal effect on bacteria but absorbed the bacteria to take it out of the body.[998]

Bentonite (mortmorsilonite) has been developed in a contemporary method, in which it absorbs the viruses through a binding process. The chemically-modified bentonite nano-particles exhibited significant reduction in three viruses: HIV-1, Influenza H3N2, and Avian Flu H5N1. It has been recommended that the clay could be used for different viral infections, in which it could be placed in cream for chickenpox or cold sores; in spermicidal gels for viral STDs; in intranasal sprays for Urbani SARS or influenza, in hand soaps for viruses; masks for healthcare workers; food supplements for viral diarrhea, adenoviruses, rotavirus; and animal feed for foot and mouth disease, bovine-shipping fever, and H5N1 in chickens.[999]

French Green Clay   Illite

* Not all French green Clays are created equal.

Possible Uses
* Arthritis, burns, detoxification, digestion, environmental protection, fatigue, food allergies, headaches, heavy metal cleanup, joints, muscular pain, radiation detox, skin problems, sore muscles, sprains
* Flesh-eating disease called buruli, salmonella[1000] caused by Mycobacterium ulcerans[1001].

Possible Benefits
* Binds mycotoxins during digestion.
* Negative electrical charge.
* Stimulates blood and lymph circulation.
* Used externally primarily but internally on occasion.

Properties
* Analgesic, anti-inflammatory, antibacterial, antimicrobial

Constituents
* Trace minerals, aluminum, calcium, cobalt, copper, dolomite, iron, manganese, magnesium, montmorillonite, phosphorous, selenium, silica, zinc, micro-algae, kelp, phytonutrients

Warning, Precautions and Side Effects
* There were two French green clays with similar mineralogy but had different effects. One killed the Buruli ulcer bacteria and the other promoted bacterial growth.[1002]

Research

In trials, they claim French clay killed up to 99 percent of superbug colonies within a 24 hour period.[1003]

Only one specific mineral, CsAg02, exhibited antibacterial activity against extended-spectrum β-lactamase (ESBL) E. coli, Escherichia coli, Mycobacterium marinum, Pseudomonas aeruginosa, Salmonella enterica serovar Typhimurium, Staphylococcus aureus, and penicillin-resistant S. aureus, Mycobacterium smegmatis, and methicillin-resistant S. aureus (MRSA).[1004]

Other Clays

- Wyoming Calcium Bentonite Clay
- Magnesium montorillonite Clay
- Sodium Bentonite montmorillonite Clay
- Zinc Bentonite montmorillonite Clay
- Hydrous Mica (Illites) similar to montmorillonite structure

Recipe

Clay facial mask

- 1/2 c. Calcium Montmorillonite clay, preferably magnesium rich, if not magnesium rich, add 1/4 c. Epsom's Salt
- 1/4 c. fulvic acid liquid or water

Scrub

- Add 1 t. baking soda or sea salt

Moisturizer
- Add 1 t. olive oil

Fango Back Mud Pack
- French (Illite), smectite (bentonite), or kaolin clay
- Optional ingredients or water
- Paint or brush onto back or arms

Optional:
- Aloe vera, chamomile, dead sea salt (mg-rich), essential oils, frankincense, fruit juice, green tea, hibiscus flower, honey, jasmine, mashed fruits/vegetables, sandalwood, seaweed, sphagnum moss (powder), sulfur, yogurt

Fango Possible Uses
- Acne[1005], bronchitis[1006], chronic dry skin[1007], dermatitis[1008], endocrine imbalance[1009], fibromyalgia[1010], immune disorders[1011], muscular pain[1012], psoriasis[1013], pulmonary tuberculosis[1014], rheumatoid arthritis[1015], osteoarthritis[1016], scars[1017]

In Conclusion, we know…

Oxygen - without it, 3 minutes and we're dead.
Water - without it, 3 days and our body starts shutting down.
Food - without it, 3 weeks and our body is starving to death.
Electrolytes: without it … soft kill.
- You get sick for a very long time and eventually die of disease.

Exercise - atrophy, use it or lose it.
- Move! Walk, stretch, breathe deeply and sweat. Start out slow if you must but start out today.

Footnotes

1   Rabe A, et al. "Learning deficit in immature rabbits with aluminum-induced neurofibrillary changes." <u>Experimental Neurology.</u> 1982, vol. 76(2), pp 441-446.

2   Petit TL, et al. "Neurofibrillary degeneration, dendritic dying back, and learning-memory deficits after aluminum administration: Implications for brain aging." <u>Experimental Neurology.</u> 1980, vol. 67(1), pp 152-162.

3   AS Kraus and WF Forbes. "Aluminum, fluoride and the prevention of Alzheimer's disease." <u>Canadian Journal of Public Health</u>. 1992, vol. 83 (2), pp 97-100.

4   Garruto RM, et al. "Imaging of calcium and aluminum in neurofibrillary tangle-bearing neurons in parkinsonism-dementia of Guam." <u>PNAS</u>. 1984, vol. 81 (6), pp 1875-1879.

5   Rifat SL, et al. "Effect of exposure of miners to aluminum powder." <u>The Lancet</u>. 1990, vol. 336 (8724), pp 1162-1165. http://www.sciencedirect.com/science/article/pii/014067369092775D

6   Garruto RM, et al. "Imaging of calcium and aluminum in neurofibrillary tangle-bearing neurons in parkinsonism-dementia of Guam." <u>PNAS</u>. 1984, vol. 81 (6), pp 1875-1879.

7   Beogman RJ and Bates LA. "Neurotoxicity of aluminum." <u>Canadian Journal of Physiology and Pharmacology</u>. 1984, vol. 62 (8), pp 1010-1014.

8   Recker RR, et al. "Evidence of aluminum absorption from the gastrointestinal tract and bone deposition by aluminum carbonate ingestion with normal renal function." <u>Journal of Laboratory and Clinical Medicine.</u> 1977, vol. 90(5), pp 810-815.

9   KG McGrath. "An earlier age of breast cancer diagnosis related to more frequent use of antiperspirants/deodorants and underarm shaving." <u>European Journal of Cancer Prevention</u>. 2003, vol. 12 (6), pp 479-485.

10   "Aluminum compounds." The Free Dictionary by Farlex. http://encyclopedia.thefreedictionary.com/aluminum

[11]   Domingo JL, et al. "Citric, malic and succinic acids as possible alternatives to deferoxamine in aluminum toxicity." <u>Clinical Toxicology</u>. 1988, vol. 26 (1-2), pp 67-79.

[12]   Rust DM and Soignet SL. "Risk/Benefit Profile of Arsenic Trioxide." <u>The Oncologist</u>. 2001, vol. 6(2), pp 29-32.

[13] Steingart R. "Managemento f patients with sickle cell disease." <u>The Medical Clinics of North America</u>. 1992, vol. 76(3), pp 669-682.

[14]   WebMD. "Arsenic Side Effects." 2005-2015. http://www.webmd.com/vitamins-supplements/ingredientmono-1226-arsenic.aspx?activeIngredientId=1226&activeIngredientName=arsenic&source=1&tabno=2

[15]   Friedrisch R, et al. "DNA damage in blood leukocytes of individuals with sickle cell disease treated with hydroxyurea" <u>Mutation Research/Genetic Toxicology and Environmental Mutagenesis</u>. 2008, vol. 649(1-2), pp 213-220.

[16]   Rust DM and Soignet SL. "Risk/Benefit Profile of Arsenic Trioxide." <u>The Oncologist</u>. 2001, vol. 6(2), pp 29-32. http://theoncologist.alphamedpress.org/content/6/suppl_2/29.full

[17] Huet, P. M.; Guillaume, E.; Cote, J.; Légaré, A.; Lavoie, P.; Viallet, A. "Noncirrhotic presinusoidal portal hypertension associated with chronic arsenical intoxication". <u>Gastroenterology</u>. 1975, vol. **68** (5 Pt 1), pp 1270–1277.

[18]   Nwachukwu CE, et al. "Antimotility agents for chronic diarrhoea in people with HIV/AIDS." <u>Cochrane HIV/AIDS Group</u>. 2008.

[19]   van Caekenberghe DL and Breyssens J. "In vitro synergistic activity between bismuth subcitrate and various antimicrobial agents against Campylobacter pyloridis (C. pylori)." <u>Antimicrob. Agents Chemother.</u> 1987, vol. 31(9), pp 1429-1430.

[20]   Turel I, et al. "Antibacterial tests of Bismuth(III)–Quinolone (Ciprofloxacin, cf) compounds against *Helicobacter pylori* and some other bacteria. Crystal structure of $(cfH_2)_2[Bi_2Cl_{10}]\cdot 4H_2O$." <u>Journal of Inorganic Biochemistry.</u> 1998, vol. 71(1-2), pp 53-60.

[21] Turel I, et al. "Antibacterial tests of Bismuth(III)–Quinolone (Ciprofloxacin, cf) compounds against *Helicobacter pylori* and some other bacteria. Crystal structure of $(cfH_2)_2[Bi_2Cl_{10}]\cdot4H_2O$." <u>Journal of Inorganic Biochemistry.</u> 1998, vol. 71(1-2), pp 53-60.

[22] Chieh-Liang Wu, et al. "Subinhibitory Bismuth-Thiols Reduce Virulence of *Pseudomonas aeruginosa*." <u>ATS Journal</u> 2002, vol. 26(6), p 731.

[23] IBID

[24] Nan Yang, et al. "Inhibition of SARS corona virus helicase by bismuth complexes." <u>Chemical Communications.</u> 2007, issue 42, pp 4413-4415..

Nan yang, et al. "Bismuth Complexes Inhibit the SARS Coronavirus." <u>Angewandte Chemie International Edition.</u> 2007, vol. 46(34), pp 6464-6468.

[25] Domenico P, et al. "Activities of Bismuth Thiols against Staphylococci and Staphylococcal Biofilms." <u>Antimicrob. Agents Chemother.</u> 2001, vol. 45(5), pp 1417-1421.

[26] Barth RF, et al. "Boron Neutron Capture Therapy of Cancer: Current Status and Future Prospects." <u>Clinical Cancer Research</u>. 2005, vol. 11, pp 3987.

[27] Nielsen FH. "Nutritional requirements for boron, silicon, vanadium, nickel, and arsenic: current knowledge and speculation." <u>The FASEB Journal</u>. 1991, vol. 5 (12), pp 2661-2667.

[28] Nielsen FH and Penland JG. "Boron supplementation of peri-menopausal women affects boron metabolism and indices associated with macromineral metabolism, hormonal status and immune function." <u>The Journal of Trace Elements in Experimental medicine</u>. 1999, vol. 12 (3), pp 251-261.

[29] RF Moseman. "Chemical disposition of boron in animals and humans." <u>Environ Health Perspect</u>. 1994, vol. 102 (7), pp 113-117.

[30] Balch, J. F., and Balch, P. A., Prescription for Nutritional Healing, 1990, pp. 17-18.

[31] Forrest Nielsen and Susan Meacham. "Growing evidence for human health benefits of boron." <u>Evidence-based Complementary Alternative Medicine</u>. 2011.

[32] Suat Çolak et al. "The neuroprotective role of boric acid on aluminum chloride-induced neurotoxicity." <u>Toxicol Ind Health</u>. 2011, vol. 27(8), pp700-710.

[33]   Newnham RE. "Essentiality of boron for healthy bones and joints." <u>Environ health Perspect.</u> 1994, vol. 102 (7), pp 83-85.

[34] Greenfelder GP. "Treatment of Fungal Infections." US Patent: US2001/0046526 A1. Date: Nov 29, 2001.

[35]   Penland JG. "Dietary boron, brain function, and cognitive performance." <u>Environ health Perspect.</u> 1994, vol. 102 (7), pp 65-72.

[36] Sobel JD, et al. "Treatment of vaginitis caused by CANDIDA GLABRATA: use of topical boric acid and flucytosine." <u>American Journal of Obstetrics & Gynecology.</u> 2003, vol. 189(5), pp 1297-1300.

[37] van Kessel K, et al. "Common Complementary and Alternative Therapies for Yeast Vaginitis and Bacterial Vaginosis: A Systematic Review." <u>Obstetrical & Gynecological Survey.</u> 2003, vol. 58(5), pp 351-358.

[38]   Palacios C. "The Role of Nutrients in Bone Health, from A to Z." <u>Critical Reviews in Food Science and Nutrition.</u> 2006, vol. 8, pp 621-628.

[39]   Penland JG. "Dietary boron, brain function, and cognitive performance." <u>Environ health Perspect</u>. 1994, vol. 102 (7), pp 65-72.

[40]   Scorei R, et al. "Comparative Effects of Boric Acid and Calcium Fructoborate on Breast Cancer Cells." <u>Biological Trace Element Research.</u> 2008, vol. 122(3), pp 197-205.

[41] Greenfelder GP. "Treatment of Fungal Infections." US Patent: US2001/0046526 A1. Date: Nov 29, 2001.

[42] De Seta F, et al. "Antifungal mechanisms supporting boric acid therapy of *Candida* vaginitis ." <u>J Antimicrob. Chemother.</u> 2009, vol. 63(2), pp 325-336.

[43] Scorei I et al. "Boron-Containing Compounds as Preventive and Chemotherapeutic Agents for Cancer." <u>Anti-Cancer Agents in Medicinal Chemistry</u>. 2010, vol. 10(4), pp 346-351.

[44]   JD Sobel and W Chaim. "Treatment of *Torulopsis glabrata* Vaginitis: Retrospective Review of Boric Acid Therapy." <u>Clin Infect Dis</u>. 1997, vol. 24 (4),pp 649-652.

45 Greenfelder GP. "Treatment of Fungal Infections." US Patent: US2001/0046526 A1. Date: Nov 29, 2001.

46 Penland JG. "Dietary boron, brain function, and cognitive performance." Environ health Perspect. 1994, vol. 102 (7), pp 65-72.

47 Kijima S, et al. "PROCESS FOR SYNTHESIS OF COENZYME Q COMPOUNDS." US Patent: 4,061,660. Date: Dec. 6, 1977.

48 Greenfelder GP. "Treatment of Fungal Infections." US Patent: US2001/0046526 A1. Date: Nov 29, 2001.

49 MJ Javid. "Topical drug for treatment and/or prevention of diabetic neuropathy, microangiopathy and diabetic and non-diabetic ulcers and wound infection." European Patent: EP2353585 A2. Date: 08/10/2010.

50 MJ Javid. "Topical drug for treatment and/or prevention of diabetic neuropathy, microangiopathy and diabetic and non-diabetic ulcers and wound infection." European Patent: EP2353585 A2. Date: 08/10/2010.

51 MJ Javid. "Topical drug for treatment and/or prevention of diabetic neuropathy, microangiopathy and diabetic and non-diabetic ulcers and wound infection." US Patent: US 2010/0222301 A1. Date: Sep 2, 2010.

52 Qureshi S, et al. "Boric acid enhances in vivo Ehrlich ascites carcinoma cell proliferation in Swiss albino mice." Toxicology. 2001, vol. 165(1), pp 1-11.

53   Penland JG. "Dietary boron, brain function, and cognitive performance." Environ health Perspect. 1994, vol. 102 (7), pp 65-72.

54 Greenfelder GP. "Treatment of Fungal Infections." US Patent: US2001/0046526 A1. Date: Nov 29, 2001.

55 Tinnell JE. "Treatment for Herpes Virus." US Patent: 4,285,934. Date: Aug 25, 1981.

56 Greenfelder GP. "Treatment of Fungal Infections." US Patent: US2001/0046526 A1. Date: Nov 29, 2001.

57 Greenfelder GP. "Treatment of Fungal Infections." US Patent: US2001/0046526 A1. Date: Nov 29, 2001.

58 RE Newnham. "Essentiality of boron for healthy bones and joints." Environ health Perspect. 1994, vol. 102 (7), pp 83-85.

59 Scorei I et al. "Boron-Containing Compounds as Preventive and Chemotherapeutic Agents for Cancer." Anti-Cancer Agents in Medicinal Chemistry. 2010, vol. 10(4), pp 346-351.

60 Penland JG. "Dietary boron, brain function, and cognitive performance." Environ Health Perspect. 1994, vol. 102 (7), pp 65-72.

61 Greenfelder GP. "Treatment of Fungal Infections." US Patent: US2001/0046526 A1. Date: Nov 29, 2001.

62 Udapudi TM. "A Clinical Study Of Borax In The Management Of Oral Candidiasis." Materia Medica. 2010

63 Travers RL, et al. "Boron and Arthritis: The Results of a Double-blind Pilot Study." Journal of Nutritional and Environmental Medicine. 1990, vol. 1 (2), pp 127-132.

64 FH Nielsen. "Studies on the relationship between boron and magnesium which possibly affects the formation and maintenance of bones." Magnesium and Trace Elements. 1990, vol. 8 (2), pp 61-69.

65 Barranco WT and Eckhert DCD. "Boric acid inhibits human prostate cancer cell proliferation." Cancer Letters. 2004, vol. 216(1-8), pp 21-29.

66 Watson-Clark RA, et al. "Model studies directed toward the application of boron neutron capture therapy to rheumatoid arthritis: Boron delivery by liposomes in rat collagen-induced arthritis." PNAS. 1998, vol. 95 (5), pp 2531-2534.

67 Penland JG. "Dietary boron, brain function, and cognitive performance." Environ Health Perspect. 1994, vol. 102 (7), pp 65-72.

68 Greenfelder GP. "Treatment of Fungal Infections." US Patent: US2001/0046526 A1. Date: Nov 29, 2001.

69 IBID

70 IBID

71 Sobel JD and Chaim W. "Treatment of TORULOPSIS GLABRATA Vaginitis: Retrospective Review of Boric Acid Therapy." Clin Infect Dis. 1997, vol. 24(4), pp 649-652.

72 IBID

73 Van Slyke KK, et al. "Treatment of vulvovaginal candidiasis with boric acid powder." American Journal of Obstetrics and Gynecology. 1981, vol. 141(2), pp 145-148.

74 Nielsen FH and Penland JG. Boron supplementation of peri-menopausal women affects boron metabolism and indices associated with macromineral metabolism, hormonal status and immune function. The Journal of Trace Elements in Experimental medicine. 1999, vol. 12 (3), pp 251-261.

75 Bhaskar CD, et al. "Boron chemicals in diagnosis and therapeutics." Future Medicinal Chemistry. 2013, vol. 5(6), pp 653-676.

76 Scorei I et al. "Boron-Containing Compounds as Preventive and Chemotherapeutic Agents for Cancer." Anti-Cancer Agents in Medicinal Chemistry. 2010, vol. 10(4), pp 346-351.

77 Greenfelder GP. "Treatment of Fungal Infections." US Patent: US2001/0046526 A1. Date: Nov 29, 2001.

78 Jacobs RT, et al. Boron-based drugs as antiprotozoals. Current Opinion in infectious Diseases. 2011, vol. 24 (6), pp 586-592.

79 Bhaskar CD, et al. "Boron chemicals in diagnosis and therapeutics." Future Medicinal Chemistry. 2013, vol. 5(6), pp 653-676.

80 Bhaskar CD, et al. "Boron chemicals in diagnosis and therapeutics." Future Medicinal Chemistry. 2013, vol. 5(6), pp 653-676.

81 Scorei I et al. "Boron-Containing Compounds as Preventive and

Chemotherapeutic Agents for Cancer." <u>Anti-Cancer Agents in Medicinal Chemistry</u>. 2010, vol. 10(4), pp 346-351.

[82] Scorei I et al. "Boron-Containing Compounds as Preventive and Chemotherapeutic Agents for Cancer." <u>Anti-Cancer Agents in Medicinal Chemistry</u>. 2010, vol. 10(4), pp 346-351.

[83] Suat Çolak et al. "The neuroprotective role of boric acid on aluminum chloride-induced neurotoxicity." <u>Toxicol Ind Health</u>. 2011, vol. 27(8), pp700-710.

[84] "Boric acid poisoning." Med. A.D.A.M. Editorial Team: David Zieve, M D, MHA, and David R. Eltz. Previously reviewed by Eric Perez, MD, Department of Emergency Medicine, St. Luke's-Roosevelt Hospital Center, New York, NY. Review provided by VeriMed Healthcare Network (2/2/2011). Updated 1/4 /2012

[85] Baker SJ, et al. "Therapeutic potential of boron-containing compounds." <u>Future Medicinal Chemistry.</u> 2009, vol. 1(7), pp 1275-1288.

[86] Jovanovic R, et al. "Antifungal agents vs. boric acid for treating chronic mycotic vulvovaginitis." <u>The Journal of Reproductive Medicine</u>. 1991, vol. 35 (8), pp 593-587.

[87] Ray D, et al. "Prevalence of CANDIDA GLABRATA and Its Response to Boric Acid Vaginal Suppositories in Comparison With Oral Fluconazole in Patients With Diabetes and Vulvovaginal Candidiasis." <u>Diabetes Care</u>. 2007, vol. 30(2), pp 312-317.

[88] Sobel JD and Chaim W. "Treatment of TORULOPSIS GLABRATA Vaginitis: Retrospective Review of Boric Acid Therapy." <u>Clin Infect Dis</u>. 1997, vol. 24(4), pp 649-652.

[89] Civigelli R, et al. "Dietary L-lysine and calcium metabolism in humans." Nutrition. 1992, vol. 8(6), pp 400-405.

[90] Evans WT and McKee DL. "ALKALI OR ALKALINE EARTH METAL OF N-BUTYRIC ACID FOR TREATMENT OF COGNITIVE AND EMOTIONAL CONDITIONS." Patent: US 6,498,247 b2. Date: Dec 24, 2002.

[91] Saito K, et al. "Widespread activation of calcium-activated neutral proteinase (calpain) in the brain in Alzheimer disease: a potential molecular basis for neuronal degeneration". <u>PNAS</u>. 1993, vol. 90 (7), pp 2628-2632.

[92] Evans WT and McKee DL. "ALKALI OR ALKALINE EARTH METAL OF N–BUTYRIC ACID FOR TREATMENT OF COGNITIVE AND EMOTIONAL CONDITIONS." Patent: US 6,498,247 b2. Date: Dec 24, 2002.

[93] Cagnacci A, et al. "Kava-Kava administration reduces anxiety in perimenopausal women." <u>Maturitas</u>. 2003, vol. 44 (2), pp 103-109.

[94] Evans WT and McKee DL. "ALKALI OR ALKALINE EARTH METAL OF N–BUTYRIC ACID FOR TREATMENT OF COGNITIVE AND EMOTIONAL CONDITIONS." Patent: US 6,498,247 b2. Date: Dec 24, 2002.

[95] Lin J, et al. "Intakes of Calcium and Vitamin D and Breast Cancer Risk in Women." <u>Arch Intern Med.</u> 2007, vol. 167(10), pp 1050-1059.

[96] Wehrens XHT, et al. FKBP12.6 "Deficiency and Defective Calcium Release Channel (Ryanodine Receptor) Function Linked to Exercise-Induced Sudden Cardiac Death." <u>Cell</u>. 2003, vol. 113 (7), pp 829-480.

[97] Evans WT and McKee DL. "ALKALI OR ALKALINE EARTH METAL OF N–BUTYRIC ACID FOR TREATMENT OF COGNITIVE AND EMOTIONAL CONDITIONS." Patent: US 6,498,247 b2. Date: Dec 24, 2002.

[98] IBID

[99] IBID

[100] Lamprecht S and Lipkin M. "Chemoprevention of colon cancer by calcium, vitamin D and folate: molecular mechanisms." <u>Nature Reviews Cancer.</u> 2003, vol. 3, pp 601-614.

[101] Evans WT and McKee DL. "ALKALI OR ALKALINE EARTH METAL OF N–BUTYRIC ACID FOR TREATMENT OF COGNITIVE AND EMOTIONAL CONDITIONS." Patent: US 6,498,247 b2. Date: Dec 24, 2002.

[102] Cagnacci A, et al. "Kava-Kava administration reduces anxiety in perimenopausal women." <u>Maturitas</u>. 2003, vol. 44 (2), pp 103-109.

[103] Evans WT and McKee DL. "ALKALI OR ALKALINE EARTH METAL OF N–BUTYRIC ACID FOR TREATMENT OF COGNITIVE AND EMOTIONAL CONDITIONS." Patent: US 6,498,247 b2. Date: Dec 24, 2002.

[104] Chapuy MC, et al. "Vitamin D_3 and Calcium to Prevent Hip Fractures in Elderly Women." <u>N Engl J Med</u>. 1992, vol. 327, pp 1637-1642.

[105]   Evans WT and McKee DL. "ALKALI OR ALKALINE EARTH METAL OF N-BUTYRIC ACID FOR TREATMENT OF COGNITIVE AND EMOTIONAL CONDITIONS." Patent: US 6,498,247 b2. Date: Dec 24, 2002.

[106]   IBID

[107]   IBID

[108]   IBID

[109]   IBID

[110]   IBID

[111]   IBID

[112]   IBID

[113]   IBID

[114]   IBID

[115]   IBID

[116]   IBID

[117]   Cagnacci A, et al. "Kava-Kava administration reduces anxiety in perimenopausal women." Maturitas. 2003, vol. 44 (2), pp 103-109.

[118]   RG Cumming. "Calcium intake and bone mass: A quantitative review of the evidence." Calcified Tissue International. 1990, vol. 47 (4), pp 194-201.

[119]   Evans WT and McKee DL. "ALKALI OR ALKALINE EARTH METAL OF N-BUTYRIC ACID FOR TREATMENT OF COGNITIVE AND EMOTIONAL CONDITIONS." Patent: US 6,498,247 b2. Date: Dec 24, 2002.

[120]   Reid IR, et al. "Effect of calcium supplementation on bone loss in postmenopausal women." The New England Journal of Medicine. 1993, vol. 328(7), pp 460-464.

121   Evans WT and McKee DL. "ALKALI OR ALKALINE EARTH METAL OF N-BUTYRIC ACID FOR TREATMENT OF COGNITIVE AND EMOTIONAL CONDITIONS." Patent: US 6,498,247 b2. Date: Dec 24, 2002.

122   IBID

123   IBID

124   IBID

125   Medical Reviewer: Williams, Robert, MD. "Calcium Deficiency: Symptoms". <u>Better Medicine from health grades</u>. 2011. http://www.localhealth.com/article/calcium-deficiency/symptoms

126   J Walleczek." Electromagnetic field effects on cells of the immune system: the role of calcium signaling." <u>FASEB Journal</u>. 1992, vol. 6 (13), pp 3177-3185.

127   Soret MG. "Antiviral activity of calcium elenolate on parainfluenza infection of hamsters." <u>Anti-Microbial Agents & Chemotherapy.</u> 1969. Pp. 160-166.

128   Carl J. Reich, MD, and Stephan Cooter, Ph.D. et. al. "Supplement to The Art of Getting Well Calcium and Vitamin D Deficiency: The Clinical Work and Theory of Carl J. Reich, MD." http://www.arthritistrust.org/Articles/Calcium%20and%20Vitamin%20D%20Deficiency.pdf

129   IBID

130   Lappe JM, et al. "Vitamin D and calcium supplementation reduces cancer risk: results of a randomized trial." <u>Am J Clin Nutr.</u> 2007, vol. 85(6), pp 1586-1591.

131   Slatopolsky E, et al. "Calcium carbonate as a phosphate binder in patients with chronic renal failure undergoing dialysis." <u>New England Journal of Medicine.</u> 1986, vol. 315(3), pp 157-161.

132   Recker RR, et al. "Effect of Estrogens and Calcium Carbonate on Bone Loss in Postmenopausal Women." <u>Ann Intern Med.</u> 1977, vol. 87(6), pp 649-655.

133   Slatopolsky E, et al. "Calcium carbonate as a phosphate binder in patients with chronic renal failure undergoing dialysis." <u>New England Journal of Medicine.</u> 1986, vol. 315(3), pp 157-161.

[134]   Slatopolsky E, et al. "Calcium carbonate as a phosphate binder in patients with chronic renal failure undergoing dialysis." <u>New England Journal of Medicine.</u> 1986, vol. 315(3), pp 157-161.

[135]   Nagbys Om Haajjika JJK, et al. "Water Chlorination and Birth Defects." <u>Epidemiology</u>. 1999 vol. 10(5).

[136]   Bing-Fang Hwang & Jouni JK Jaakkila. "Water Chlorination and Birth Defects: A Systematic Review and Meta-Analysis." <u>Archives of Environmental Health: An International Journal</u>. 2003, Vol 58(2).

[137]   http://www.radiationdetoxification.com

[138]   Wang J, Zhang L, and Sten M. "Administration of Aerosolized Terbutaline and Budesonide Reduces Chlorine Gas-Induced Acute Lung Injury." <u>Journal of Trauma-Injury Infection & Critical Care</u>. 2004, vol. 56(4), pp 850-862

[139]   June K. Dunnick and Ronald L. Melnick. Assessment of the Carcinogenic Potential of Chlorinated Water: Experimental Studies of Chlorine, Chloramine, and Trihalomethanes. <u>Journal of National Cancer Institute.</u> 1993. Vol 85(10), pp 817-822.

[140]   Bove F, Shim Y, and Zeitz P. "Drinking water contaminants and adverse pregnancy outcomes: a review." <u>Environmental Health Perspectives</u>. 2002. Vol 110(1): pp 61-74.

[141]   Eaton JW, Kolpin CF, et al. "Chlorinated Urban Water: A Cause of Dialysis-Induced Hemolytic Aemia." <u>Science</u>. 1974, vol. 181 (4098), pp 463-464.

[142]   Smith QR and Rapoport SI. "Carrier-mediated transport of chloride across the blood-brain barrier." <u>J Neurochem.</u> 1984, vol. 42(3), pp 754-763.

[143]   Matthias F. Heinitz. "Alzheimer's Disease and Trace Elements: Chromium and Zinc." <u>Journal of Orthomolecular Medicine.</u> 2005, vol. 20(2), pp 89-92.

[144]   MA Alim Al-Bari, et al. "*In vitro* Antimicrobial Properties and Cytotoxic Activities of (Two Novel Deleted) Chromium Complexes." <u>Research Journal of Agriculture and Biological Sciences</u>. 2007, vol. 3 (6), pp 599-604.

[145]   IBID

[146]   Schroeder HA, et al. "Chromium deficiency as a factor in atherosclerosis." Journal of Chronic Disease. 1970, vol. 23 (2), pp 123-142.

[147] Yoshimoto S, et al. "Effect of chromium administration on glucose tolerance in stroke-prone spontaneously hypertensive rats with streptozotocin-induced diabetes." Metabolism. 1992, vol. 41(6), pp 636-642.

[148]   Matthias F. Heinitz. "Alzheimer's Disease and Trace Elements: Chromium and Zinc." Journal of Orthomolecular Medicine. 2005, vol. 20(2), pp 89-92.

[149]   MA Alim Al-Bari, et al. "*In vitro* Antimicrobial Properties and Cytotoxic Activities of (Two Novel Deleted) Chromium Complexes." Research Journal of Agriculture and Biological Sciences. 2007, vol. 3 (6), pp 599-604.

[150]   Yu-Rong Tang, et al. "Studies of five microelement contents in human serum, hair, and fingernails correlated with aged hypertension and coronary heart disease." Biological Trace Element Research. 2003, vol. 92(2), pp 97-103.

[151]   RA Anderson. "CHROMIUM IN THE PREVENTION AND CONTROL OF DIABETES." Diabetes and Metabolism. 2000, vol. 26, pp 22-27.

[152]   Pattar GR, et al. "Chromium picolinate positively influences the glucose transporter system via affecting cholesterol homeostasis in adipocytes cultured under hyperglycemic diabetic conditions." Mutation Research/Genetic Toxicology and Environmental Mutagenesis. 2006, vol. 610(1-2), pp 93-100.

[153]   IBID

[154] Yoshimoto S, et al. "Effect of chromium administration on glucose tolerance in stroke-prone spontaneously hypertensive rats with streptozotocin-induced diabetes." Metabolism. 1992, vol. 41(6), pp 636-642.

[155]   Mertz W. "Chromium in human nutrition: a review." Journal of Nutrition. 1993, vol. 123(4).

[156]   R Donnelly and A Garber. "Diabetes, Obesity and Metabolism." Endocrinology & Metabolism. 2011, vol. 44 p 122.

[157]   MA Alim Al-Bari, et al. "*In vitro* Antimicrobial Properties and Cytotoxic Activities of (Two Novel Deleted) Chromium Complexes." Research Journal of Agriculture and Biological Sciences. 2007, vol. 3 (6), pp 599-604.

[158]   RA Anderson. "CHROMIUM IN THE PREVENTION AND CONTROL OF DIABETES." Diabetes and Metabolism. 2000, vol. 26, pp 22-27.

[159]   MA Alim Al-Bari, et al. "*In vitro* Antimicrobial Properties and Cytotoxic Activities of (Two Novel Deleted) Chromium Complexes." Research Journal of Agriculture and Biological Sciences. 2007, vol. 3 (6), pp 599-604.

[160]   R Donnelly and A Garber. "Diabetes, Obesity and Metabolism." Endocrinology & Metabolism. 2011, vol. 44 p 122.

[161]   Arora R, etal. "Estimation of serum zinc and copper in children with acute diarrhea." Biological Trace Element Research. 2006, vol. 114(1-3), PP 121-126.

[162]   Inestrosa NC, et al. "Copper brain homeostasis: Role of amyloid precursor protein and prion protein." IUBMB Life. 2005, vol. 57 (9), pp 645-650.

[163]   MD Tilson. "Decreased Hepatic Copper Levels A Possible Chemical Marker for the Pathogenesis of Aortic Aneurysms in Man." Arch Surg. 1982, vol. 117 (9), pp 1212-1213.

[164]   M Olivares and R Uauy. "Copper as an essential nutrient." Am J Clin Nutr. 1996, vol. 63 (5), pp 791S-796S.

[165]   Horie M, et al. "Inactivation and morphological changes of avian influenza virus by copper ions." Archives of Virology. 2008, vol. 153 (8), pp 1467-1472.

[166]   Jonas J, et al. "Impaired Mechanical Strength of Bone in Experimental Copper Deficiency." Annals of Nutrition and Metabolism. 1993, vol. 37 (5), pp 245-252.

[167]   Daniel KG, et al. "Clioquinol and pyrrolidine dithiocarbamate complex with copper to form proteasome inhibitors and apoptosis inducers in human breast cancer cells." Breast Cancer Research. 2005, vol. 7, pp R897-R908.

[168] Weissman z, et al. "The high copper tolerance of CANDIDA ALBICANS is mediated by a P-type ATPase." PNAS. 2000, vol97(7), pp 3520-3525.

[169]   Higdon J, et al. Micronutrient Information Center. Linus Pauling Institute. Oregon State University. 2012.

[170]   Higdon J, et al. "Micronutrient Information Center." Linus Pauling Institute. Oregon State University. 2012.

[171]   Arora R, etal. "Estimation of serum zinc and copper in children with acute diarrhea." <u>Biological Trace Element Research.</u> 2006, vol. 114(1-3), PP 121-126.

[172]   Olivares M and Uauy R. "Copper as an essential nutrient." <u>Am J Clin Nutr</u>. 1996, vol. 63 (5), pp 791S-796S.

[173]   Gaggelli E, et al. "Copper Homeostasis and Neurodegenerative Disorders (Alzheimer's, Prion, and Parkinson's Diseases and Amyotrophic Lateral Sclerosis)." <u>Chem Rev.</u> 2006, vol. 106, pp 1995-2044.

[174]   Higdon J, et al. Micronutrient Information Center. Linus Pauling Institute. Oregon State University. 2012.

[175]   Inestrosa NC, et al. "Copper brain homeostasis: Role of amyloid precursor protein and prion protein." <u>IUBMB Life.</u> 2005, vol. 57 (9), pp 645-650.

[176]   Adsule S, et al. "Novel Schiff Base Copper Complexes of Quinoline-2 Carboxaldehyde as Proteasome Inhibitors in Human Prostate Cancer Cells." <u>J Med Chem.</u> 2006, vol. 49(24), pp 7242-7246.

[177]   Yazar M, et al. "Synovial fluid and plasma selenium, copper, zinc, and iron concentrations in patients with rheumatoid arthritis and osteoarthritis." <u>Biological Trace Element Research.</u> 2005, vol. 106(2), pp 123-132.

[178]   Sen CK, et al. "Copper-induced vascular endothelial growth factor expression and wound healing." <u>AJP.</u> 2002, vol. 282(5), pp H1821-H1827.

[179]   Griffith DP, et al. "Acquired Copper Deficiency: A Potentially Serious and Preventable Complication Following Gastric Bypass Surgery." <u>Obesity (Silver Spring).</u> 2009, vol. 17 (4), pp 827-831.

[180]   WR Walker and DM Keats. "An investigation of the therapeutic value of the 'copper bracelet'-dermal assimilation of copper in arthritic/rheumatoid conditions." <u>Agents and Actions.</u> 1976, vol. 6 (4), pp 454-459.

[181]   Higdon J, et al. Micronutrient Information Center. Linus Pauling Institute. Oregon State University. 2012.

[182]   Earl S. Ford. "Serum Copper Concentration and Coronary Heart Disease among US Adults." <u>Am J Epidemiol</u>. 2000, vol. 151 (12), pp 1182-1188.

[183]   Dhanarajan Shanthakumari, et al. "Effect of fluoride intoxication on lipidperoxidation and antioxidant status in experimental rats". <u>Toxicology</u>. 2004, vol. 204 (2-3), pp 219-228.

[184]   Elizabeth Frerrell, CPDH, "Masters in Dental Hygiene." <u>Truly Alive magazine</u>. September/October 2009, p.11.

[185]   Bernstein DS, et al. "Prevalence of Osteoporosis in High- and Low-Fluoride Areas in North Dakota." <u>JAMA</u>. 1966, vol. 198 (5), pp 499-504.

[186]   Riggs BL, et al. "EFFECT OF FLUORIDE TREATMENT ON THE FRACTURE RATE IN POSTMENOPAUSAL WOMEN WITH OSTEOPOROSIS." <u>New England Journal of Medicine.</u> 1990, vol. 322(12), pp 802-809.

[187]   www.mednat.org/cancro/nacci_english.pdf

[188]   Susheela AK, et al. "Excess fluoride ingestion and thyroid hormone derangements in children living in Delhi, India" <u>Fluoride</u>. 2005, vol. 38 (2), pp 98-108.

[189]   Li XS, Zhi JL, and Gao RO. "Effects of fluoride exposure on intelligence in children." <u>Fluoride</u>. 1994, vol. 28 (4), pp 189-192.

[190]   AS Kraus and WF Forbes. "Aluminum, fluoride and the prevention of Alzheimer's disease." <u>Canadian Journal of Public Health</u>. 1992, vol. 83 (2), pp 97-100.

[191]   Danielson C, et al. "Hip Fractures and Fluoridation in Utah's Elderly Population". <u>JAMA</u>. 1992, vol. 268 (6), pp 746-748.

[192]   Jochen Klaus, et al. "Bones and Crohn's: No benefit of adding sodium fluoride or ibandronate to calcium and vitamin D." <u>World J Gastroenterol</u>. 2011, vol. 17 (3), pp 334-342.

[193]   www.mednat.org/cancro/nacci_english.pdf

[194]   Riggs BL, et al. "EFFECT OF FLUORIDE TREATMENT ON THE FRACTURE RATE IN POSTMENOPAUSAL WOMEN WITH OSTEOPOROSIS." <u>New England Journal of Medicine.</u> 1990, vol. 322(12), pp 802-809.

[195]   Sandra Goodman. "Therapeutic effects of organic Germanium." <u>Medical Hypotheses</u>. 1988, vol. 26 (3), pp 207-215.

[196] SA Levine and PM Kidd. "Oxygen-Nutrition for Super Health Research Breakthrough on an Oxygen Catalyst". <u>Journal of Orthomolecular Medicine</u>. Vol 1 (3), pp 145-148.

[197] IBID

[198] Sandra Goodman. "Therapeutic effects of organic Germanium." <u>Medical Hypotheses</u>. 1988, vol. 26 (3), pp 207-215.

[199] IBID

[200] SA Levine and PM Kidd. "Oxygen-Nutrition for Super Health Research Breakthrough on an Oxygen Catalyst". <u>Journal of Orthomolecular Medicine</u>. Vol 1 (3), pp 145-148.

[201] IBID

[202] IBID

[203] IBID

[204] IBID

[205] Shu-Wen Jao, et al. Effect of germanium on 1, 2-dimethylhydrazine-induced intestinal cancer in rats. Diseases of the Colon & Rectum. 1990, vol. 33 (2), pp 99-104.

[206] SA Levine and PM Kidd. "Oxygen-Nutrition for Super Health Research Breakthrough on an Oxygen Catalyst". <u>Journal of Orthomolecular Medicine</u>. Vol 1 (3), pp 145-148.

[207] IBID

[208] IBID

[209] Zhang Z, et al. "Influence of germanium on PGE of rat with rheumatoid arthritis." <u>Journal of Pharmaceutical Practice.</u> 2009-3.

[210] Sandra Goodman. "Therapeutic effects of organic Germanium." <u>Medical Hypotheses</u>. 1988, vol. 26 (3), pp 207-215.

[211] IBID

[212]   SA Levine and PM Kidd. "Oxygen-Nutrition for Super Health Research Breakthrough on an Oxygen Catalyst". Journal of Orthomolecular Medicine. Vol 1 (3), pp 145-148.

[213]   Sandra Goodman. "Therapeutic effects of organic Germanium." Medical Hypotheses. 1988, vol. 26 (3), pp 207-215.

[214]   Zhang Z, et al. "Influence of germanium on PGE of rat with rheumatoid arthritis." Journal of Pharmaceutical Practice. 2009-3.

[215]   Chuang-Hao Lin, et al. Germanium dioxide induces mitochondria-mediated apoptosis in Neuro-2A cells. NeuroToxicology. 2006, vol. 27 (6), pp 1052=1063.

[216]   Suzuki F, Brutkiewicz RR, and Pollard RB. Ability of sera from mice treated with Ge-132, compound, to inhibit experimental murine ascites tumours. Br J Cancer. 1985, vol. 52 (5), pp 757-763.

[217]   Goodman, S. "Therapeutic effects of organic Germanium." Medical Hypotheses. Vol 26, Issue 3, 1988, pp. 207-215.

[218]   Chuang-Hao Lin, et al. "Germanium dioxide induces mitochondria-mediated apoptosis in Neuro-2A cells." NeuroToxicology. 2006, vol. 27 (6), pp 1052=1063.

[219]   Goodman, S. "Therapeutic effects of organic Germanium." Medical Hypotheses. Vol 26, Issue 3, 1988, pp. 207-215.

[220]   IBID

[221]   IBID

[222]   IBID

[223]   Kamijo M, et al. "[An autopsy case of chronic germanium intoxication presenting peripheral neuropathy, spinal ataxia, and chronic renal failure]." Rinsho Shinkeigaku. 1991, vol. 31(2), pp 191-196.

[224]   Goodman, S. "Therapeutic effects of organic Germanium." Medical Hypotheses. Vol 26, Issue 3, 1988, pp. 207-215.

[225]   Dr. Kazuhiko Asai. Miracle Cure: Organic Germanium
http://www.internationalsunrise.com/new/download/Miracle_Cure_-
_Organic_Germanium_--_Kazuhiko_Asai_PhD.pdf

[226]   Tannenbreg K, et al. "Nucleic Acid Aptamers as novel class of Therapeutics to mitigate Alzheimer's Disease Pathology." Current Alzheimer Research. 2013, vol. 10(4), pp 442-448(7).

[227] Danscher G and Larsen A. "Effects of dissolucytotic gold ions on recovering brain lesions." Histochem Cell Biol. 2010, vol. 133, pp 367.

[228]   IBID

[229]   Paciotti GF, et al. "Colloidal Gold: A Novel Nanoparticle Vector for Tumor Directed Drug Delivery." Drug Delivery. 2004,m vol. 11(3), pp 169-183.

[230]   Richards DG et al. "Gold and its relationship to Neurological/glandular conditions." International Journal of Neuroscience. 2002, vol. 112(1), pp 31-53.

[231] Gray SJ, et al. "Liver function studies in diabetes mellitus." Ann Intern Med. 1946, vol. 24(1), pp 72-79.

[232] Hrushikesh MJ, et al. "Gold Nanoparticles as carriers for efficient transmucosal insulin delivery." Langmuir. 2006, vol. 22(1), pp 300-305.

[233]   Abraham GE and Himmel PB. "Management of Rheumatoid Arthritis: Rational for the Use of Colloidal Metallic Gold." Journal of Nutritional and Environmental Medicine. 1997, vol. 7(4), pp 295-305.

[234] Yong-Tang Wang, et al. "The use of a gold nanoparticle-based adjuvant to improve the therapeutic efficacy of hNgR-Fc protein immunization in spinal cord-injured rats." Biomaterials. 2011, vol. 32(31), pp 7988-7998.

[235] Danscher G and Larsen A. "Effects of dissolucytotic gold ions on recovering brain lesions." Histochem Cell Biol. 2010, vol. 133, pp 367.

[236]   F Delange. "Iodine deficiency as a cause of brain damage." Postgrad Med J. 2001, vol. 77 pp 217-220.

[237]   Teng W, et al. "Effect of Iodine Intake on Thyroid Diseases in China." New England Journal of Medicine. 2006, vol. 354, pp 2783-2793.

238   Hiroomi Funahashi, et al. "Seaweed Prevents Breast Cancer?" <u>Cancer Science</u>. 2001, vol. 92 (5), pp 483-487.

239   Vermiglio F, et al. "Defective Neuromotor and Cognitive Ability in Iodine-Deficient Schoolchildren of an Endemic Goiter Region in Sicily." <u>Journal of Clinical Endocrinology & Metabolism</u>. 1990, vol. 79 (2), pp 379-384.

240   IBID

241   IBID

242   Teng W, et al. "Effect of Iodine Intake on Thyroid Diseases in China." <u>New England Journal of Medicine.</u> 2006, vol. 354, pp 2783-2793.

243   Delange F. "Neonatal Screening for Congenital Hypothyroidism Results and Perspectives." <u>Horm Res</u>. 1997, vol. 48, pp 51-61.

244   Vermiglio F, et al. "Defective Neuromotor and Cognitive Ability in Iodine-Deficient Schoolchildren of an Endemic Goiter Region in Sicily." <u>Journal of Clinical Endocrinology & Metabolism</u>. 1990, vol. 79 (2), pp 379-384.

245   C Aceves and B Anguiano. "Chap. 6. Is Iodine an Antioxidant and Antiproliferative Agent for the Mammary and Prostate Glands?" VR Preedy, et al. <u>Comprehensive Handbook of Iodine: Nutritional, Biochemical, Pathological and Therapeutic Aspects</u>. 2009.Academic Press, Elsevier. MA

246   Teng W, et al. "Effect of Iodine Intake on Thyroid Diseases in China." <u>New England Journal of Medicine.</u> 2006, vol. 354, pp 2783-2793.

247   IBID

248   F Delange. "Iodine deficiency as a cause of brain damage." <u>Postgrad Med J.</u> 2001, vol. 77 pp 217-220.

249   IBID

250   Zanzonico PB and Becker DV. "Effects of Time of Administration and Dietary Iodine Levels on Potassium Iodide (Ki) Blockade of Thyroid Irradiation By 131I From Radioactive Fallout." <u>Health Physics</u>. 2000, vol. 78 (6), pp 660-667.

[251] Konofal E, et al. "Iron Deficiency in Children With Attention-Deficit/Hyperactivity Disorder." <u>Arch Pediatr Adolesc Med</u>. 2004, vol. 158 (12), pp 113-115.

[252] Kirkpatrick CH, et al. "Inhibition of Growth of *Candida albicans* by Iron-Unsaturated Lactoferrin: Relation to Host-Defense Mechanisms in Chronic Mucocutaneous Candidiasis." <u>J Infect Dis.</u> 1971, vol. 124(6), pp 539-544.

[253] Auerbach M, et al. "Intravenous Iron Optimizes the Response to Recombinant Human Erythropoietin in Cancer Patients With Chemotherapy-Related Anemia: A Multicenter, Open-Label, Randomized Trial ." <u>JCO</u> 2004, vol. 22(7), pp 1301-1307.

[254] Sang-Chol Lee, et al. "Iron Supplementation Inhibits Cough Associated With ACE Inhibitors." <u>Hypertension.</u> 2001, vol. 38, pp 166-170.

[255] Verdon F, et al. "Iron supplementation for unexplained fatigue in non-anaemic women: double blind randomised placebo controlled trial." <u>BMJ</u> 2003, vol. 326, p 1124.

[256] Zimmermann MB and Köhrle J. "The Impact of Iron and Selenium Deficiencies on Iodine and Thyroid Metabolism: Biochemistry and Relevance to Public Health." <u>Thyroid.</u> 2002, vol. 12(10), pp 867-878.

[257] Walter T, et al. "Effect of mild iron deficiency on infant mental development scores." <u>Journal of Pediatrics</u>. 1983, vol. 102 (4), pp 519-522.

[258] Silverberg DS, et al. "Intravenous iron for the treatment of predialysis anemia." <u>Kidney International.</u> 1999, vol. 55, pp S79-S85.

[259] Scholl TO. "Iron status during pregnancy: setting the stage for mother and infant." <u>Am J Clin Nutr.</u> 2005, vol. 81(5), pp 1218S-1222S.

[260] O'Keeffe ST, Gavin K and Lavan JN. "Iron Status and Restless Legs Syndrome in the Elderly." <u>Age and Aging.</u> 1994, vol. 23(3), pp 200-203.

[261] Neil Gordon. "Iron deficiency and the intellect." <u>Brain and Development</u>. 2003, vol. 25 (1), pp 3-8.

[262] Patruta SI and HÖRL WH. "Risks and Side Effects of Iron Therapy." 1999, vol. 55, pp S125-S130.

263 Zimmermann MB and Köhrle J. "The Impact of Iron and Selenium Deficiencies on Iodine and Thyroid Metabolism: Biochemistry and Relevance to Public Health." <u>Thyroid.</u> 2002, vol. 12(10), pp 867-878.

264 John L. Beard. "Iron Deficiency and Brain Function." Department of Nutrition, The Pennsylvania State University, University Park, PA, 16802, USA.
11th International Symposium on Trace Elements in Man and Animals   Abstracts jn.nutrition.org at NIH Lib Acquisitions Unit/MSC 1150 on August 20, 2008

265 Viteri FE, et al. "The Consequences of Iron Deficiency and Anaemia in Pregnancy on Maternal Health, the Foetus and the Infant." <u>SCN News</u>. Vol 11. Maternal and Child Nutrition. UNSSCN. 1994, p 76.

266 IBID

267 Patruta SI and HÖRL WH. Risks and Side Effects of Iron Therapy. 1999, vol. 55, pp S125-S130.

268 IBID

269 IBID

270 Weinberg ED. "Iron, infection and sudden infant death." <u>Medical Hypotheses</u>. 2001, vol. 56(6), pp 731-734.

271 Stevens RG, et al. "Body iron stores and the risk of cancer." <u>New England Journal of Medicine.</u> 1988, vol. 319(16), pp 1047-1052.

272 Nelson RL. "Iron and Colorectal Cancer Risk: Human Studies." <u>Nutrition Revciews.</u> 2001, vol. 59(5), pp 140-148.

273 Zecca L, et al. "Iron, brain ageing and neurodegenerative disorders." <u>Nature Reviews Neuroscience.</u> 2004, vol. 5, pp 863-873.

274 Bullen JJ and Rogers HJ. "Bacterial Iron Metabolism and Immunity to *Pasteurella septica* and *Escherichia coli*." <u>Nature.</u> 1969, vol. 224, pp 380-382.

275 Weinberg ED. "Iron, infection, and neoplasia." <u>Clinical Physiology and Biochemistry.</u> 1986, vol. 4(1), pp 50-60.

276 Walker EM Jr. and Walker SM. "Effects of iron overload on the immune system." <u>Ann Clin Lab Sci.</u> 2000, vol. 30(4), pp 354-365.

277   Balch, J. F. and Balch, P. A. Prescription for Nutritional Healing, 1990, p.20.

278 Nunes PV, et al. "Lithium and risk for Alzheimer's disease in elderly patients with bipolar disorder." British Journal of Psychiatry. 2007, vol. 190, pp 359-360.

279 Fornai F, et al. "Lithium delays progression of amyotrophic lateral sclerosis." PNAS 2007, vol. 105(6), pp 2052-2057.

280 Simhandl C and Mersch J. "Lithium and bipolar disorder--a renaissance?" Neuroopsychiatr. 2007, vol. 21(2), pp 121-130.

281 Wroblewski BA, et al. "Effectiveness of valproic acid on destructive and aggressive behaviours in patients with acquired brain injury." Brain Injury. 1997, vol. 11(1), pp 37-48.

282 Jihong Xu, et al. "Chronic Treatment With a Low Dose of Lithium Protects the Brain Against Ischemic Injury by Reducing Apoptotic Death." Stroke. 2003, vol. 34, pp 1287-1292.

283 Nunes PV, et al. "Lithium and risk for Alzheimer's disease in elderly patients with bipolar disorder." British Journal of Psychiatry. 2007, vol. 190, pp 359-360.

284 Leung-Wah Yick, et al. "Lithium Chloride Reinforces the Regeneration-Promoting Effect of Chondroitinase ABC on Rubrospinal Neurons after Spinal Cord Injury." Journal of Neurotrauma. 2004, vol. 21(7), pp 932-943.

285 Zarse K, et al. "Low-dose lithium uptake promotes longevity in humans and metazoans." European Journal of Nutrition. 2011, vol. 50(5), pp 387-389.

286 Jihong Xu, et al. "Chronic Treatment With a Low Dose of Lithium Protects the Brain Against Ischemic Injury by Reducing Apoptotic Death." Stroke. 2003, vol. 34, pp 1287-1292.

 Moore GJ, et al. "Lithium increases *N*-acetyl-aspartate in the human brain: in vivo evidence in support of bcl-2's neurotrophic effects?" Biological Psychiatry. 2000, vol. 48(1), pp 1-8.

287 Nunes PV, et al. "Lithium and risk for Alzheimer's disease in elderly patients with bipolar disorder." British Journal of Psychiatry. 2007, vol. 190, pp 359-360.

288 Mendelson J, et al. "Serum Magnesium in Delirium Tremens and Alcoholic Hallucinosis." J of Nervous & Mental Disease. 1959, vol. 128(4), pp 352-357.

[289]   EB Rink. "Magnesium Deficiency in Alcoholism." <u>Alcoholism: Clinical and Experimental Research</u>. 1986, vol. 10 (6), pp 590-594.

[290]   Cohen L and Kitzes R. "Magnesium sulfate in the treatment of variant angina." <u>Magnesium</u>. 1984, vol. 3 (1), pp 46-49.

[291]   Poleszak E, et al. "Antidepressant- and anxiolytic-like activity of magnesium in mice." <u>Phamacology Biochemistry and Behavior</u>. 2004, vol. 78 (1), pp 7-12.

[292]   Speziale G, et al. "Arrhythmia prophylaxis after coronary artery bypass grafting: regimens of magnesium sulfate administration. Thoracic and Cardiovascular Surgeon. 2000, vol. 48 (1), pp 22-26.

[293]   Saris N-EL, et al. "Magnesium: An update on physiological, clinical and analytical aspects." <u>Clinica Chimica Acta.</u> 2000, vol. 294(1-2), pp 1-26.

[294]   Saris N-EL, et al. "Magnesium: An update on physiological, clinical and analytical aspects." <u>Clinica Chimica Acta.</u> 2000, vol. 294(1-2), pp 1-26.

[295]   Huntsman RG, Hurn BAL and Lehmann H. "OBSERVATIONS ON THE EFFECT OF MAGNESIUM ON BLOOD COAGULATION." <u>J Clin Pathol.</u> 1960, vol. 13, pp 99-101.

[296]   Jee SHa, et al. "The effect of magnesium supplementation on blood pressure: a meta-analysis of randomized clinical trials." <u>American Journal of Hypertension.</u> 2002, vol. 15(8), pp 691-696.

[297]   Saris N-EL, et al. "Magnesium: An update on physiological, clinical and analytical aspects." <u>Clinica Chimica Acta.</u> 2000, vol. 294(1-2), pp 1-26.

[298]   Freedman AM, et al. "Magnesium deficiency-induced cardiomyopathy: Protection by vitamin E." <u>Biochemical and Biophysical Research Communications</u>. 1990, vol. 179 (3), pp 1102-1106.

[299]   IM Cox, et al. "Red blood cell magnesium and chronic fatigue syndrome." <u>The Lancet</u>. 1991, vol. 337 (8744), pp 757-760.

[300]   Winkler AW, Smith PK and Hoff HE. "INTRAVENOUS MAGNESIUM SULFATE IN THE TREATMENT OF NEPHRITIC CONVULSIONS IN ADULTS." <u>J Clin Invest.</u> 1942, vol. 21(2), pp 207-216.

[301]   Gamelin L, et al. "Prevention of Oxaliplatin-Related Neurotoxicity by Calcium and Magnesium Infusions A Retrospective Study of 161 Patients Receiving Oxaliplatin Combined with 5-Fluorouracil and Leucovorin for Advanced Colorectal Cancer." <u>Clin Cancer Res</u>. 2004, vol. 10, p 4055.

[302]   Gottlieb SS, et al. "Prognostic importance of the serum magnesium concentration in patients with congestive heart failure." <u>Journal of the American College of Cardiology</u>. 1990, vol. 16 (4), pp 827-831.

[303]   Teragawa H, et al. "The Preventive Effect of Magnesium on Coronary Spasm in Patients With Vasospastic Angina." <u>Chest Journal.</u> 2000, vol. 118(6), pp 1690-1695.

[304]   Poleszak E, et al. "Antidepressant- and anxiolytic-like activity of magnesium in mice. <u>Phamacology Biochemistry and Behavior</u>. 2004, vol. 78 (1), pp 7-12.

[305]   Lopez-Ridaura R, et al. "Magnesium Intake and Risk of Type 2 Diabetes in Men and Women." <u>Diabetes Care</u>. 2004, vol. 27 (1), pp 134-140.

[306]   Saris N-EL, et al. "Magnesium: An update on physiological, clinical and analytical aspects." <u>Clinica Chimica Acta.</u> 2000, vol. 294(1-2), pp 1-26.

[307]   Leaver DD, et al. "NEUROLOGICAL CONSEQUENCES OF MAGNESIUM DEFICIENCY: CORRELATIONS WITH EPILEPSY." 1987, vol. 14 (5), pp 361-370.

[308]   Ronald J Grisanti. "Is Your Patient's Teenager at Risk of Dying from Heart Failure? What Every Parent MUST Know to Prevent Sudden Death!" <u>Magnes Res</u>. 1993, vol. 6 (2), pp 191-192.

[309]   IBID

[310]   Abraham GE and Flechas JD. "Management of Fibromyalgia: Rationale for the Use of Magnesium and Malic Acid." <u>Journal of Nutritional and Environmental Medicine</u>. 1992, vol. 3 (1), pp 49-59.

[311]   Gaspar AZ, et al. "The Influence of Magnesium on Visual Field and Peripheral Vasospasm in Glaucoma." <u>Ophthalomologica</u>. 1995, vol. 209 (1), pp 11-13,

[312]   Gordin A, et al. "Magnesium: A New Therapy for Idiopathic Sudden Sensorineural Hearing Loss." <u>Otology & Neurotology</u>. 2002, vol. 23 (4), pp 447-451.

[313] Ueshima K. "Magnesium and ischemic heart disease: a review of epidemiological, experimental, and clinical evidences." Magnesium Research. 2005, vol. 18(4), pp 275-284.

[314] Jones JE, et al. "Magnesium metabolism in hyperthyroidism and hypothyroidism". J Clin Invest. 1966, vol. 45 (6), pp 891-900.

[315] Cockburn F, et al. "Neonatal convulsions associated with primary disturbance of calcium, phosphorus, and magnesium metabolism." Archives of Disease in Childhood. 1973, vol. 49, p 99.

[316] IBID

[317] Saris N-EL, et al. "Magnesium: An update on physiological, clinical and analytical aspects." Clinica Chimica Acta. 2000, vol. 294(1-2), pp 1-26.

[318] Ueshima K. "Magnesium and ischemic heart disease: a review of epidemiological, experimental, and clinical evidences." Magnesium Research. 2005, vol. 18(4), pp 275-284.

[319] MF McCarty. "Magnesium taurate and fish oil for prevention of migraine." Medical Hypotheses. 1996, vol. 47 (6), pp 461-466.

[320] Bobkowski W, et al. "The importance of magnesium status in the pathophysiology of mitral valve prolapse." Magnesium Research. 2005, vol. 18 (1), pp 35-52.

[321] Cockburn F, et al. "Neonatal convulsions associated with primary disturbance of calcium, phosphorus, and magnesium metabolism." Archives of Disease in Childhood. 1973, vol. 49, p 99.

[322] Attias J, et al. "Oral magnesium intake reduces permanent hearing loss induced by noise exposure." American Journal of Otolaryngology. 1994, vol. 15 (1), pp 26-32.

[323] Sahota O, et al. "Vitamin D insufficiency and the blunted PTH response in established osteoporosis: the role of magnesium deficiency." Osteoporosis International. 2006, vol. 17 (7), pp 1013-1021.

[324] Witlin AG and Baha MS. "Magnesium sulfate therapy in preeclampsia and eclampsia." Obstetrics & Gynecology. 1998, vol. 92 (5), pp 883-889.

[325] Ronald J Grisanti. "Is Your Patient's Teenager at Risk of Dying from Heart Failure? What Every Parent MUST Know to Prevent Sudden Death!" <u>Magnes Res.</u> 1993, vol. 6 (2), pp 191-192.

[326] Thwaites CL, et al. "Magnesium sulphate for treatment of severe tetanus: a randomised controlled trial." <u>Lancet.</u> 2006, vol. 368(9545), pp 1436-1443.

[327] Teragawa H, et al. "The Preventive Effect of Magnesium on Coronary Spasm in Patients With Vasospastic Angina." <u>Chest Journal.</u> 2000, vol. 118(6), pp 1690-1695.

[328] Ronald J Grisanti. "Is Your Patient's Teenager at Risk of Dying from Heart Failure? What Every Parent MUST Know to Prevent Sudden Death!" <u>Magnes Res.</u> 1993, vol. 6 (2), pp 191-192..

[329] Walker AF, et al. "Magnesium Supplementation Alleviates Premenstrual Symptoms of Fluid Retention." <u>Journal of Women's Health.</u> 2009, vol. 7(9), pp 1157-1165.

[330] http://curezone.com/art/read.asp?ID=33&db=8&C0=16

[331] Magnesium (Mg). Mosby's Medical Dictionary, 8th edition. # SYMBOL 211 \f "Symbol" \s 10#2009, Elsevier. http://medical-dictionary.thefreedictionary.com/magnesium

[332] MAGNESIUM DEFICIENCY & SUDDEN DEATH, Written and Researched by Ronald J. Grisanti D.C., D.A.B.C.O. http://curezone.com/art/read.asp?ID=33&db=8&C0=16

[333] Abbott. "Magnesium Sulfate." The Comprehensive resource for physicians, drug and illness information. RxMed. http://www.rxmed.com/b.main/b2.pharmaceutical/b2.1.monographs/CPS-%20Monographs/CPS-%20(General%20Monographs-%20M)/MAGNESIUM%20SULFATE.html

[334] Poleszak E, et al. "Antidepressant- and anxiolytic-like activity of magnesium in mice." <u>Phamacology Biochemistry and Behavior</u>. 2004, vol. 78 (1), pp 7-12.

[335] IBID

[336] Cohen L and Kitzes R. "Magnesium sulfate in the treatment of variant angina." <u>Magnesium.</u> 1984, vol. 3 (1), pp 46-49.

[337] Marx AJ. "Formulations of Magnesium Compounds for Local Application and Methods of Treatment using the same." US Patent 5,898,037. Date: Apr 27, 1999.

[338] Edmundas Širvinskas and Rokas Laurinaitis. "Use of magnesium sulfate in anesthesiology." Medicina. 2002, vol. 38(7), pp 695-698.

[339] Marx AJ. "Formulations of Magnesium Compounds for Local Application and Methods of Treatment using the same." US Patent 5,898,037. Date: Apr 27, 1999.

[340] Mahajan P, et al. "Comparison of nebulized magnesium sulfate plus albuterol to nebulized albuterol plus saline in children with acute exacerbations of mild to moderate asthma." J of Emergency Medicine. 2004, vol. 27(1), pp 21-25.

[341] Fox M. "CORRECTED: Epsom salt can prevent cerebral palsy: U.S. study." Reuters. 2008. http://www.reuters.com/article/2008/01/31/us-palsy-salt-correction-idUSHUN17633820080131?sp=true

[342] Marx AJ. "Formulations of Magnesium Compounds for Local Application and Methods of Treatment using the same." US Patent 5,898,037. Date: Apr 27, 1999.

[343] Leor J and Kloner RA. "An experimental model examining the role of magnesium in the therapy of acute myocardial infarction." Am J of Cardiology. 1995, vol. 75(17), pp 1292-1293.

[344] Marx AJ. "Formulations of Magnesium Compounds for Local Application and Methods of Treatment using the same." US Patent 5,898,037. Date: Apr 27, 1999.

[345] IBID

[346] IBID

[347] IBID

[348] GA Eby and KL Eby. "Rapid recovery from major depression using magnesium treatment." Medical Hypotheses. 2006, vol. 67 (2), pp 362-370.

[349] Epsom Salts to Detox, Relieve Pain: The Health and Beauty Benefits of Magnesium Sulfate | Suite101.com http://elaine-moore.suite101.com/epsom-salts-a47574#ixzz1oN2odwWd

350 Walker AF, et al. "Magnesium Supplementation Alleviates Premenstrual Symptoms of Fluid Retention." Journal of Women's Health. 2009, vol. 7(9), pp 1157-1165.

351 Muthuswamy Anantharaman, et al. "β-Amyloid Mediated Nitration of Manganese Superoxide Dismutase : Implication for Oxidative Stress in a APP[NLh/NLh] X PS-1[P264L/P264L] Double Knock-In Mouse Model of Alzheimer's Disease." The American Journal of Pathology. 2006, vol. 168 (5), pp 1608-1618.

352 Robinson BH. "The role of manganese superoxide dismutase in health and disease." J of Inherited metabolic Disease. 1998, vol. 21(5), pp 598-603.

353 Hung RJ, et al. "Genetic polymorphisms of *MPO, COMT, MnSOD, NQO1*, interactions with environmental exposures and bladder cancer risk." Carcinogenesis. 2004, vol. 25 (6), pp 973-978.

354 Leach RM Jr., et al. "Studies on the role of manganese in bone formation: II. Effect upon chondroitin sulfate synthesis in chick epiphyseal cartilage." Archives of Biochemistry and Biophysics. 1969, vol. 133(1), pp 22-28.

355 Takeda A. "Manganese action in brain function." Brain Research Reviews. 2003, vol. 41(1), pp 79-87.

356 Li JJ, et al. "Phenotypic changes induced in human breast cancer cells by overexpression of manganese-containing superoxide dismutase." Oncogene. 1995, vol. 10 (10), 1989-2000.

357 Robinson BH. "The role of manganese superoxide dismutase in health and disease." J of Inherited metabolic Disease. 1998, vol. 21(5), pp 598-603.

358 Day BJ. "Catalytic antioxidants: a radical approach to new therapeutics." Drug Discovery Today. 2004, vol. 9(13), pp 557-566.

359 Kim GW, et al. "Manganese Superoxide Dismutase Deficiency Exacerbates Cerebral Infarction After Focal Cerebral Ischemia/Reperfusion in Mice Implications for the Production and Role of Superoxide Radicals." Stroke. 2002, vol. 33, pp 809-815.

360 Yongmin Liu, et al. MnSOD inhibits proline oxidase-induced apoptosis in colorectal cancer cells. Carcinogenesis. 2005, vol. 25 (8), pp 1335-1342.

361 Treiber N, et al. "The role of manganese superoxide dismutase in skin aging." Dermatoendocrinol. 2012, vol. 4(3), pp 232-235.

[362] Bertera S, et al. "Gene Transfer of Manganese Superoxide Dismutase Extends Islet Graft Function in a Mouse Model of Autoimmune Diabetes." Diabetes. 2003, vol. 52(2), pp 387-393.

[363] Takeda A. "Manganese action in brain function." Brain Research Reviews. 2003, vol. 41(1), pp 79-87.

[364] Day BJ. "Catalytic antioxidants: a radical approach to new therapeutics." Drug Discovery Today. 2004, vol. 9(13), pp 557-566.

[365] Keller JN, et al. "Mitochondrial Manganese Superoxide Dismutase Prevents Neural Apoptosis and Reduces Ischemic Brain Injury: Suppression of Peroxynitrite Production, Lipid Peroxidation, and Mitochondrial Dysfunction." J of Neruoscience. 1998, vol. 18(2), pp 687-697.

[366] Day BJ. "Catalytic antioxidants: a radical approach to new therapeutics." Drug Discovery Today. 2004, vol. 9(13), pp 557-566.

[367] Liang LP, et al. "Mitochondrial superoxide production in kainate-induced hippocampal damage." Neuroscience. 2000, vol. 101(3), pp 563-570.

[368] Treiber N, et al. "The role of manganese superoxide dismutase in skin aging." Dermatoendocrinol. 2012, vol. 4(3), pp 232-235.

[369] LW Oberley. "Mechanism of the tumor suppressive effect of MnSOD over expression." Biomedicine & Pharmacotherapy. 2005, vol. 59 (4), pp 143-148.

[370] IBID

[371] WC Dougall and HS Nick. "Manganese Superoxide Dismutase: A Hepatic Acute Phase Protein Regulated by Interleukin-6 and Glucocorticoids." Endocrinology. 1991, vol. 129 (5), pp 2376-2384.

[372] Woodson K, et al. "Manganese superoxide dismutase (MnSOD) polymorphism, α-tocopherol supplementation and prostate cancer risk in the Alpha-Tocopherol, Beta-Carotene Cancer Prevention Study (Finland)." Cancer Causes & Control. 2003, vol. 14(6), pp 513-518.

[373] Aschner JL and Aschner M. "Nutritional aspects of manganese homeostasis." Molecular Aspects of Medicine. 2005, vol. 26(4-5), pp 353-362.

[374] "Therapeutic Uses of Molybdenum." International Molybdenum Association. http://www.imoa.info/HSE/environmental_data/human_health/molybdenum_therapeutic_uses.php

[375] IBID

[376] IBID

[377] IBID

[378] IBID

[379] IBID

[380] Li JY. "Epidemiology of esophageal cancer in China." National Cancer Institute Monograph. 1982, vol. 62, pp 113-11120.

[381] Lozak A, et al. "Determination of chromium, selenium, and molybdenum in a therapeutic diet." Die Pharmazie-An International Journal of Pharmaceutical Sciences. 2004, vol. 59 (11), pp 824-827 (4).

[382] "Therapeutic Uses of Molybdenum." International Molybdenum Association. http://www.imoa.info/HSE/environmental_data/human_health/molybdenum_therapeutic_uses.php

[383] IBID

[384] Lozak A, et al. Determination of chromium, selenium, and molybdenum in a therapeutic diet. Die Pharmazie-An International Journal of Pharmaceutical Sciences. 2004, vol. 59 (11), pp 824-827 (4).

[385] "Therapeutic Uses of Molybdenum." International Molybdenum Association. http://www.imoa.info/HSE/environmental_data/human_health/molybdenum_therapeutic_uses.php

[386] IBID

[387] IBID

[388] IBID

[389] Al-Omar MA, et al. "Role of Molybdenum Hydroxylases in Disease." Saudi Pharmaceutical Journal. 2005, vol. 13(1), pp 1-13.

[390] Metz JA, Anderson JJ and Gallagher PN Jr. "Intakes of calcium, phosphorus, and protein, and physical-activity level are related to radial bone mass in young adult women." Am J Clin Nutr. 1993, vol. 58(4), pp 537-542.

[391] Leonard Sax. The Institute of Medicine's "Dietary Reference Intake" for Phosphorus: A Critical Perspective. J Am Coll Nutr. 2001, vol. 20 (4), pp 271-278.

[392] IBID

[393] Draper HH, Sie T-L, and Bergan JG. "Osteoporosis in Aging Rats Induced by High Phosphorus Diets." J Nutr. 1972, vol. 102, pp 1133-1142.

[394] Reynolds EC. "Anticariogenic complexes of amorphous calcium phosphate stabilized by casein phosphopeptides: A review." Special Care in Dentistry.1998, vol. 18(1), pp 8-16.

[395] Moe SM. "Disorders Involving Calcium, Phosphorus, and Magnesium." Primary Care: Clinics in Office Practice. 2008, vol. 35(2), pp 215-237.

[396] Wendy Brooks. "Calcium Phosphorus Balance." 5/18/2012.
http://www.marvistavet.com/html/calcium_phosphorus_balance.html

[397] Sally Squires. "The Amazing Statistics and Dangers of Soda Pop." Washington Post. 2/27/2001, p HE 10.
http://www.americanchiropractic.net/general_%20interest/Statistics%20and%20 Dangers%20of%20Soda%20.pdf

[398] "What is the optimal serum potassium level in cardiovascular patients?" J Am Coll Cardiol. 2004, vol. 43 (2), pp 155-161.

[399] Cooke RE, et al. "THE EXTRARENAL CORRECTION OF ALKALOSIS ASSOCIATED WITH POTASSIUM DEFICIENCY." J Clin Invest. 1952, vol. 31 (8), pp 798-805.

[400] Garrow JS. "Loss of Brain Potassium." The Lancet. 1967, vol. 290 (7517), pp 643-645.

[401] Pelaia G, et al. "Potential role of potassium channel openers in the treatment of asthma and chronic obstructive pulmonary disease." Life Sciences. 2002, vol. 70(9), pp 977-990.

[402] Tannen RL. "Effects of Potassium on Blood Pressure Control." <u>Ann Intern Med.</u> 1983, vol. 98(5_Part_2), pp 773-780.

[403] "What is the optimal serum potassium level in cardiovascular patients?" <u>J Am Coll Cardiol.</u> 2004, vol. 43 (2), pp 155-161.

[404] Pelaia G, et al. "Potential role of potassium channel openers in the treatment of asthma and chronic obstructive pulmonary disease." <u>Life Sciences.</u> 2002, vol. 70(9), pp 977-990.

[405] Greene DA and Lattimer SA. "Impaired rat sciatic nerve sodium-potassium adenosine triphosphatase in acute streptozocin diabetes and its correction by dietary myo-inositol supplementation." <u>J Clin Invest.</u> 1983, vol. 72(3), pp 1058-1063.

[406] Ernst JP, Doose H, Baier WK. "Bromides were effective in intractable epilepsy with generalized tonic-clonic seizures and onset in early childhood." <u>Brain Dev.</u> 1988, vol. 10 (6), pp 385-388

[407] "What is the optimal serum potassium level in cardiovascular patients?" <u>J Am Coll Cardiol.</u> 2004, vol. 43 (2), pp 155-161.

[408] Knochel JP. "Heat stroke and related heat stress disorders." <u>DM</u> 1989, vol. 35(5), pp 301-377.

[409] "What is the optimal serum potassium level in cardiovascular patients?" <u>J Am Coll Cardiol.</u> 2004, vol. 43 (2), pp 155-161.

[410] Tannen RL. "Effects of Potassium on Blood Pressure Control." <u>Ann Intern Med.</u> 1983, vol. 98(5_Part_2), pp 773-780.

[411] Garrow JS. Loss of Brain Potassium. The Lancet. 1967, vol. 290 (7517), pp 643-645.

[412] Johnson CJ, Peterson DR and Smith EK. "Myocardial tissue concentrations of magnesium and potassium in men dying suddenly from ischemic heart disease." <u>Am J Clin Nutr.</u> 1979, vol. 32(5),., pp 967-970.

[413] Chandra P, et al. "Correlation of total body potassium and leukemic cell mass in patients with chronic lymphocytic leukemia." <u>Blood.</u> 1975, vol. 5e (4), pp 594-603.

414   Garrow JS. "Loss of Brain Potassium." <u>The Lancet</u>. 1967, vol. 290 (7517), pp 643-645.

415   Beeton C and Chandy KG. "Potassium Channels, Memory T Cells, and Multiple Sclerosis." <u>Neuroscientist</u>. 2005, vol. 11 (6), pp 550-562.

416   Bonaccorsi A, et al. "Mechanism of Potassium Relaxation of Arterial Muscle." <u>Blood Vessels.</u> 1977, vol. 14, pp 261-276.

417   Horvath B, et al. *"Muscular Dystrophy. Cation Concentrations in Residual Muscle."* <u>Journal of Applied Physiology</u>. 1955, vol. 8 (1), pp 22-30.

418   Maclennan WJ, et al. "IS WEAKNESS IN OLD AGE DUE TO MUSCLE WASTING?" <u>Age and Ageing.</u> 1980, vol. 9(3), pp 188-192.

419   Xueyou Hu, et al. "KCa1.1 Potassium Channels Regulate Key Proinflammatory and Invasive Properties of Fibroblast-like Synoviocytes in Rheumatoid Arthritis." <u>Journal of Biological Chemistry</u>. 2012, vol. 287, pp 4014-4022.

420   Ding EL and Mozaffarian D. "Optimal Dietary Habits for the Prevention of Stroke." <u>Semin Neurol.</u> 2006, vol. 26(1), pp 011-023.

421   Garrow JS. "Loss of Brain Potassium." <u>The Lancet</u>. 1967, vol. 290 (7517), pp 643-645.

422   Ernst JP, Doose H, Baier WK. "Bromides were effective in intractable epilepsy with generalized tonic-clonic seizures and onset in early childhooD." <u>Brain Dev.</u> 1988, vol. 10 (6), pp 385-388

423   Dr. Chase's Recipes Information for Everybody, 1888, Stanton and Van Vliet Co., Chicago. http://books.google.com/books?id=LVMYAAAAMAAJ&pg=PA14&dq=dr+chases+r ecipe+1888&hl=en&sa=X&ei=MpyMT7z0DOiLiAK9jJHKCA&ved=0CDYQ6AEwAA#v =onepage&q&f=false

424   Brad M Dworkin. "Selenium deficiency in HIV infection and the acquired immunodeficiency syndrome (AIDS)". <u>Chemico-Biological Interactions</u>. 1994, vol. 91 (2-3), pp 181-186.

[425] Ishrat T, et al. "Selenium prevents cognitive decline and oxidative damage in rat model of streptozotocin-induced experimental dementia of Alzheimer's type." <u>Brain Research.</u> 2009, vol. 1281, pp117-127.

[426] Helzlouer KJ, et al. "Selenium, Lycopene, α-Tocopherol, β-Carotene, Retinol, and Subsequent Bladder Cancer." <u>Cancer Res.</u> 1989, vol. 49, p 6144.

[427] Ya-Jun Hu, et al. "The protective role of selenium on the toxicity of cisplatin-contained chemotherapy regimen in cancer patients." <u>Biological Trace Element Research.</u> 1997, vol. 56(3), pp 331-341.

[428] Watrach AM, et al." Inhibition of human breast cancer cells by selenium." <u>Cancer Letters.</u> 1984, vol. 25 (1), pp 41=47.

[429] PD Whanger. "Selenium and its relationship to cancer: an update." <u>British Journal of Nutrition.</u> 2004, vol. 91 (1), pp 11-28.

[430] Boyne R and Arthur JR. "The response of selenium-deficient mice to Candida albicans infection." <u>Journal of Nutrition.</u> 1986, vol. 116(5), pp 816-822.

[431] Fleming CR, et al. "Selenium deficiency and fatal cardiomyopathy in a patient on home parenteral nutrition." <u>Gastroenterology.</u> 1982, vol. 83(3), pp 689-693.

[432] Bleys J, et al. "Serum selenium levels and all-cause, cancer, and cardiovascular mortality among US adults." <u>Arch Intern Med</u>. 2008, vol. 168(4), pp 404-410.

[433] TR Shearer and LL David. "Role of calcium in selenium cataract." <u>Current Eye Research</u>. 1982, vol. 2 (11), pp 777-784.

[434] Shamberger RJ, et al. "Antioxidants and Cancer. I. Selenium in the Blood of Normals and Cancer Patients." <u>JNCI</u> 1073, vol. 50(4), pp 863-870.

[435] Ishrat T, et al. "Selenium prevents cognitive decline and oxidative damage in rat model of streptozotocin-induced experimental dementia of Alzheimer's type." <u>Brain Research.</u> 2009, vol. 1281, pp117-127.

[436] Finley JW, et al. Selenium from High Selenium Broccoli Protects Rats from Colon Cancer." <u>J Nutr</u>. 2000, vol. 130 (9), 2384-2389.

[437] G Kine & L Watson. "Colorectal Cancer Protective Effects and the Dietary Micronutrients Folate, Methionine, Vitamins B6, B12, C, E, Selenium, and Lycopene." <u>Nutrition and Cancer</u>. 2006, vol. 56 (1), pp 11-21.

[438]   Dworkin B, et al. "Low blood selenium levels in patients with cystic fibrosis compared to controls and healthy adults." JPEN J Parenter Enteral Nutr. 1987, vol. 11 (1), pp 38-41.

[439] Mustafa Naziroglu. "Role of Selenium on Calcium Signaling and Oxidative Stress-induced Molecular Pathways in Epilepsy." Neurochemical Research. 2009, vol. 34(12), pp 2181-2191.

[440]   Melinda A. Beck. "Selenium Deficiency Increases the Risk of Viral Infections." University of North Carolina Chapel Hill, Chapel Hill, NC.
11th International Symposium on Trace Elements in Man and Animals   Abstracts jn.nutrition.org at NIH Lib Acquisitions Unit/MSC 1150 on August 20, 2008

[441] Wasantwisut E. "Nutrition and development: other micronutrients' effect on growth and cognition." The Southeast Asian Journal of Tropical Medicine and Public Health. 1997, vol. 28(2), pp 78-82.

[442]   Shammmberger RJ, et al. "Antioxidants and Cancer. I. Selenium in the Blood of Normals and Cancer Patients." J Natl Cancer Inst. 1973, vol. 50 (4), pp 863-870.

[443]   Shu Yu Yu, et al. "Protective role of selenium against hepatitis B virus and primary liver cancer in Qidong." Biological Trace Elements Research. 1997, vol. 56 (1), pp 117-124.

[444] Shamberger RJ, et al. "Antioxidants and Cancer. I. Selenium in the Blood of Normals and Cancer Patients." JNCI 1073, vol. 50(4), pp 863-870.

[445] Hatfield DL. Beck MA. "Selenium as an antiviral agent." Selenium. Kluwer Academic Publishers. 2001, Chapter 19, pp 1-2

[446]   Shammmberger RJ, et al. "Antioxidants and Cancer. I. Selenium in the Blood of Normals and Cancer Patients." J Natl Cancer Inst. 1973, vol. 50 (4), pp 863-870.

[447] Batist G. "Selenium Preclinical Studies of Anticancer Therapeutic Potential." Biological Trace Element Research. Humana Press Inc. 1988, pp 223-224.
http://link.springer.com/chapter/10.1007/978-1-4612-4606-0_17#page-1

[448] Soullier BK, et al. "Effect of selenium on azoxymethane-induced intestinal cancer in rats fed high fat diet." Cancer Letters. 1981, vol. 12(4), pp 343-348.

[449]   Suadicani P, et al. "Serum selenium concentration and risk of ischaemic heart disease in a prospective cohort study of 3000 males." Atherosclerosis. 1992, vol.

96(1), pp 33-42.

[450]   Hatfield DL. Beck MA. "Selenium as an antiviral agent." Selenium. <u>Kluwer Academic Publishers</u>. 2001, Chapter 19, pp 1-2.

[451]   Manary MJ, et al. "Selenium status, kwashiorkor and congestive heart failure." <u>Acta Paediatrica</u>. 2001, vol. 90(8), pp 950-952.

[452]   Shu Yu Yu, et al. "Protective role of selenium against hepatitis B virus and primary liver cancer in Qidong." <u>Biological Trace Elements Research</u>. 1997, vol. 56 (1), pp 117-124.

[453] Knekt P, et al. "Serum Selenium and Subsequent Risk of Cancer Among Finnish Men and Women." <u>JNCI</u> 1990, vol. 82(10), pp 864-868.

[454] Rederstorff M, et al. "Understanding the importance of selenium and selenoproteins in muscle function." <u>Cellular and Molecular Life Sciences</u>. 2006, vol. 63(1), pp 52-59.

[455] Hatfield DL. Beck MA. "Selenium as an antiviral agent." Selenium. Kluwer Academic Publishers. 2001, Chapter 19, pp 1-2

[456] Nikam S, et al. "Oxidative stress in Parkinson's disease." <u>Indian Journal of Clinical Biochemistry.</u> 2009, vol. 24(1), pp 98-101.

[457]   Clark, et al. "Decreased incidence of prostate cancer with selenium supplementation: results of a double-blind cancer prevention trial." <u>British Journal of Urology</u>. 1998, vol. 81 (5), pp 730-734.

[458]   Knekt P, et al. "Serum Selenium, Serum Alpha-Tocopherol, and the Risk of Rheumatoid Arthritis." <u>Epidemiology</u>. 2000, vol. 11 (4), pp 402-405.

[459]   Kharaeva Z, et al. "Clinical and biochemical effects of coenzyme Q_{10}, vitamin E, and selenium supplementation to psoriasis patients." <u>Nutrition.</u> 2009, vol. 25(3), pp 295-302.

[460] Knekt P, et al. "Serum Selenium and Subsequent Risk of Cancer Among Finnish Men and Women." <u>JNCI</u> 1990, vol. 82(10), pp 864-868.

[461]   Virtamo Jarmo, et al. "SERUM SELENIUM AND THE RISK OF CORONARY HEART DISEASE AND STROKE." <u>Am J Epidemiol.</u> 1985, vol. 122(2), pp 276-282.

[462]   Rhead WJ, et al. "The vitamin E and selenium status of infants and the sudden infant death syndrome." <u>Bioinorganic Chemistry.</u> 1972, vol. 1(4), pp 289-294.

[463] Thorling EB, Overvad K, and Bjerring P. "ORAL SELENIUM INHIBITS SKIN REACTIONS TO UV LIGHT IN HAIRLESS MICE." Acta Pathologica Microbiologica Scandinavica Series A: Pathology. 1983, vol. 91A (1-6), pp 81-84.

[464] Alissa EM, et al. "The controversy surrounding selenium and cardiovascular disease: a review of the evidence." Medical Science Monitor: International Medical Journal of Experimental and Clinical Research. 2003, vol. 9 (1), pp RA9-18.

[465] Hatfield DL. Beck MA. "Selenium as an antiviral agent." Selenium. Kluwer Academic Publishers. 2001, Chapter 19, pp 1-2.

[466] Zeng H and Combs Jr GF. "Selenium as an anticancer nutrient: roles in cell proliferation and tumor cell invasion." The Journal of Nutritional Biochemistry. 2008, vol. 19(1), pp 1-7.

[467] IBID

[468] Batist G. "Selenium Preclinical Studies of Anticancer Therapeutic Potential." Biological Trace Element Research. Humana Press Inc. 1988, pp 223-224.

[469] Zeng H and Combs Jr GF. "Selenium as an anticancer nutrient: roles in cell proliferation and tumor cell invasion." The Journal of Nutritional Biochemistry. 2008, vol. 19(1), pp 1-7.

[470] IBID

[471] Hatfield DL. Beck MA. "Selenium as an antiviral agent." Selenium. Kluwer Academic Publishers. 2001, Chapter 19, pp 1-2

[472] Zeng H and Combs Jr GF. "Selenium as an anticancer nutrient: roles in cell proliferation and tumor cell invasion." The Journal of Nutritional Biochemistry. 2008, vol. 19(1), pp 1-7.

[473] IBID

[474] IBID

[475] Flores-Mateo G, et L. "Selenium and coronary heart disease: a meta-analysis." Am J Clin Nutr. 2006, vol. 84(4), pp 762-773.

[476] Jenkins KJ, et al. "PREVENTION OF NUTRITIONAL MUSCULAR DYSTROPHY IN CALVES AND LAMBS BY SELENIUM AND VITAMIN E ADDITIONS TO THE MATERNAL MINERAL SUPPLEMENT." <u>Canadian Journal of Animal Science</u>. 1974, vol. 54 (1), pp 49-60.

[477] TR Shearer and LL David. "Role of calcium in selenium cataract." <u>Current Eye Research</u>. 1982, vol. 2 (11), pp 777-784.

[478] Flores-Mateo G, et al. "Selenium and coronary heart disease: a meta-analysis." <u>Am J Clin Nutr.</u> 2006, vol. 84(4), pp 762-773.

[479] Szarka CE, et al. "Chemoprevention of cancer." <u>Current Problems in Cancer</u>. 1994, vol. 18 (1), pp 6-79.

[480] Mark Stengler, The Natural Physician's Healing Therapies, 2010, Prentice Hall Press, p 417

[481] Chidsey CA III, Kahn G. "Methods and Solutions for Treating Male Pattern Alopecia." US Patent 4,596,812. Date: June 24, 1986.

[482] Klaus Schwarz. "SILICON, FIBRE, AND ATHEROSCLEROSIS." <u>The Lancet</u>. 1977, vol. 309 (8009), pp 454-457.

[483] Jugdaohsingh R, et al. "Dietary Silicon Intake Is Positively Associated With Bone Mineral Density in Men and Premenopausal Women of the Framingham Offspring Cohort." <u>JBMR</u> 2004, vol. 19(2), pp 297-307.

[484] Carlisle EM. "Silicon: A requirement in bone formation independent of vitamin D." <u>Calcified Tissue International.</u> 1981, vol. 33(1), pp 27-34.

[485] Pérez-Granados AM and Vaquero MP. "Silicon, aluminum, arsenic and lithium: essentiality and human health implications." <u>Journal of Nutrition</u>. Health & Aging. 2002, vol. 6 (2), pp 154-162.

[486] IBID

[487] IBID

[488] Jugdaohsingh R, et al. "Dietary Silicon Intake Is Positively Associated With Bone Mineral Density in Men and Premenopausal Women of the Framingham Offspring Cohort." <u>JBMR</u> 2004, vol. 19(2), pp 297-307.

[489]   Satadal Das, et al. "Role of silicon in modulating the internal morphology and growth of *Mycobacterium tuberculosis*." <u>Indian Journal of Tuberculosis</u>. 2000, vol. 47 (2), pp 87-91.

[490]   Klaus Schwarz. "SILICON, FIBRE, AND ATHEROSCLEROSIS." <u>The Lancet</u>. 1977, vol. 309 (8009), pp 454-457.

[491]   Lipworth L, et al. "Silicone Breast Implants and Connective Tissue Disease: An Updated Review of the Epidemiologic Evidence." <u>Annals of Plastic Surgery.</u> 2004, vol. 52(6), pp 598-601.

[492]   Jugdaohsingh R, et al. "Dietary Silicon Intake Is Positively Associated With Bone Mineral Density in Men and Premenopausal Women of the Framingham Offspring Cohort." <u>JBMR</u> 2004, vol. 19(2), pp 297-307.

[493]   Birchall JD and Chappell JS. "The chemistry of aluminum and silicon in relation to Alzheimer's disease." <u>Clinical Chemistry.</u> 1988, vol. 34(2), pp 265-267.

[494]   Edith Muriel Carlisle. "Silicon as a trace nutrient." <u>Science of The Total Environment.</u> 1988, vol. 73 (1-2), p 95-106.

[495]   Lara HH, et al. "Silver Nan particles are broad-spectrum bactericidal and virucidal compounds." <u>Journal of Nanobiotechnology.</u> 2010, vol. 9(30), p 1-8.

[496]   Xingmao Jiang, et al. "Aerosol Method for Nano silver-silica Composite Anti-microbial Agent." US Patent US 2009/0175948 A1. Date: Jul. 9, 2009.

[497]   Singh M, et al. "Nanotechnology in Medicine and Antibacterial Effect of Silver Nanoparticles." <u>Digest Journal of Nanomaterials and Biostructures.</u> 2008, vol. 3(3), pp 115-122.

[498]   Xingmao Jiang, et al. "Aerosol Method for Nano silver-silica Composite Anti-microbial Agent." US Patent US 2009/0175948 A1. Date: Jul. 9, 2009.

[499]   Hee Sun Park, et al. "Attenuation of allergic airway inflammation and hyperresponsiveness in a murine model of asthma by silver nanoparticles." <u>Int J Nanomedicine.</u> 2010, vol. 5, pp 505-515.

[500]   Xingmao Jiang, et al. "Aerosol Method for Nano silver-silica Composite Anti-microbial Agent." US Patent US 2009/0175948 A1. Date: Jul. 9, 2009.

[501] Ki-Young Yoon, et al. "Antimicrobial Characteristics of Silver Aerosol Nanoparticles against *Bacillus subtilis* Bioaerosols." Environmental Engineering Science. 2008, vol. 25(2), pp 289-294.

[502] Xingmao Jiang, et al. "Aerosol Method for Nano silver-silica Composite Anti-microbial Agent." US Patent US 2009/0175948 A1. Date: Jul. 9, 2009.

[503] IBID

[504] IBID

[505] IBID

[506] Singh M, et al. "NANOTECHNOLOGY IN MEDICINE AND ANTIBACTERIAL EFFECT OF SILVER NANOPARTICLES." Digest Journal of Nanomaterials and Biostructures. 2008, vol. 3(3), pp 115-122.

[507] Saravanan S, et a.. "Preparation, characterization and antimicrobial activity of a bio-composite scaffold containing chitosan/nano-hydroxyapatite/nano-silver for bone tissue engineering" International Journal of Biological Macromolecules. 2011, vol. 49(2), pp 188-193.

[508] Yezhelyev MV, et al. "Emerging use of nanoparticals in diagnosis and treatment of breast cancer." The Lancet Oncology. 2006, vol. 7(8), pp 657-667.

[509] Ha Ryong Kim, et al. "Genotoxic effects of silver Nan particles stimulated by oxidative stress in human normal bronchial epithelial (BEAS-2B) cells." Mutation Research/Genetic Toxicology and Environmental Mutagenesis. 2011, vol. 726(2), pp 129-135.

[510] Jin-Sook Hyun, et al. "Effects of repeated silver nanoparticles exposure on the histological structure and mucins of nasal respiratory mucosa in rats." Toxicology Letters. 2008, vol. 182(1-3), pp 24-228.

[511] Xingmao Jiang, et al. "Aerosol Method for Nano silver-silica Composite Anti-microbial Agent." US Patent US 2009/0175948 A1. Date: Jul. 9, 2009.

[512] Arora S, et al. "Cellular responses induced by silver Nan particles: In vitro studies." Toxicology Letters. 2008, vol. 179920, PP 93-100.

[513] Singh M, et al. "Nanotechnology in Medicine and Antibacterial Effect of Silver Nanoparticles." Digest Journal of Nanomaterials and Biostructures. 2008, vol. 3(3), pp 115-122.

[514]   Panacek A, et al. "Antifungal activity of silver nanoparticles against Candida spp." <u>Biomaterials.</u> 2009, vol. 30(31), pp 6333-6340.

[515]   nanda M and Saravanan M. "Biosynthesis of silver nanoparticles from *Staphylococcus aureus* and its antimicrobial activity against MRSA and MRSE." <u>Nanomedicine: Nanotechnology, Biology and Medicine.</u> 2009, vol. 5(4), pp 452-456.

[516]   Pimentel RC, et al. "Silver Nanoparticles Nanocarriers, Synthesis and Toxic Effect on Cervical Cancer Cell Lines." <u>BioNano Science.</u> 2013, vol. 3(2), pp 198-207.

[517]   Jingfeng Tang, et al. "Rapid and simultaneous detection of *Ureaplasma parvum* and *Chlamydia trachomatis* antibodies based on visual protein microarray using gold nanoparticles and silver enhancement." <u>Diagnostic Microbiology and Infectious Disease</u>. 2010, vol. 67(2), pp 122-128.

[518]   Xingmao Jiang, et al. "Aerosol Method for Nano silver-silica Composite Anti-microbial Agent." US Patent US 2009/0175948 A1. Date: Jul. 9, 2009.

[519]   Jin-Sook Hyun, et al. "Effects of repeated silver nanoparticles exposure on the histological structure and mucins of nasal respiratory mucosa in rats." <u>Toxicology Letters.</u> 2008, vol. 182(1-3), pp 24-228.

[520]   Xingmao Jiang, et al. "Aerosol Method for Nano silver-silica Composite Anti-microbial Agent." US Patent US 2009/0175948 A1. Date: Jul. 9, 2009.

[521]   Fortina P, et al. "Applications of nanoparticles to diagnostics and therapeutics in colorectal cancer." <u>Trends in Biotechnology.</u> 2007, vol. 25(4), pp 145-152.

[522]   Xingmao Jiang, et al. "Aerosol Method for Nano silver-silica Composite Anti-microbial Agent." US Patent US 2009/0175948 A1. Date: Jul. 9, 2009.

[523]   IBID

[524]   IBID

[525]   V Edwards-Jones. "The benefits of silver in hygiene, personal care and healthcare." <u>Letters in Applied Microbiology.</u> 2009, vol. 49(2), pp 147-152.

[526] Holladay RJ, Christensen H, and Moeller WD. "Treatment of Humans with Colloidal Silver Composition." US Patent US 7,135,195 B2. Date: Nov 14, 2006.

[527] Xingmao Jiang, et al. "Aerosol Method for Nano silver-silica Composite Anti-microbial Agent." US Patent US 2009/0175948 A1. Date: Jul. 9, 2009.

[528] Vora P. "NANO SILVER INDUCED STEM CELL ACTIVATION." http://www.space-age.com/StemCellGelPhotoGallery.pdf

[529] Xingmao Jiang, et al. "Aerosol Method for Nano silver-silica Composite Anti-microbial Agent." US Patent US 2009/0175948 A1. Date: Jul. 9, 2009.

[530] Sondi I, Salopek-Sondi B. "Silver Nan particles as antimicrobial agent: a case study on E. coli as a model for Gram-negative bacteria." Journal of Colloid and Interface Science. 2004, vol. 275 (1), pp 177-182.

[531] Holladay RJ, Christensen H, and Moeller WD. "Treatment of Humans with Colloidal Silver Composition." US Patent US 7,135,195 B2. Date: Nov 14, 2006.

[532] Xingmao Jiang, et al. "Aerosol Method for Nano silver-silica Composite Anti-microbial Agent." US Patent US 2009/0175948 A1. Date: Jul. 9, 2009.

[533] Holladay RJ, Christensen H, and Moeller WD. "Treatment of Humans with Colloidal Silver Composition." US Patent US 7,135,195 B2. Date: Nov 14, 2006.

[534] IBID

[535] IBID

[536] Xingmao Jiang, et al. "Aerosol Method for Nano silver-silica Composite Anti-microbial Agent." US Patent US 2009/0175948 A1. Date: Jul. 9, 2009.

[537] Holladay RJ, Christensen H, and Moeller WD. "Treatment of Humans with Colloidal Silver Composition." US Patent US 7,135,195 B2. Date: Nov 14, 2006.

[538] Nanda M and Saravanan M. "Biosynthesis of silver nanoparticles from *Staphylococcus aureus* and its antimicrobial activity against MRSA and MRSE." Nanomedicine: Nanotechnology, Biology and Medicine. 2009, vol. 5(4), pp 452-456.

[539] Xingmao Jiang, et al. "Aerosol Method for Nano silver-silica Composite Anti-microbial Agent." US Patent US 2009/0175948 A1. Date: Jul. 9, 2009.

[540] IBID

[541] V Edwards-Jones. "The benefits of silver in hygiene, personal care and healthcare." Letters in Applied Microbiology. 2009, vol. 49(2), pp 147-152.

[542] Panacek A, et al. "Silver Colloid Nanoparticles: Synthesis, Characterization, and Their Antibacterial Activity." The Journal of Physical Chemistry. 2006, vol. 110 (33), pp 16248-16253.

[543] IBID

[544] Elechiguerra J, et al. "Interaction of silver nanoparticles with HIV-1." BioMed Central Ltd. 2005
http://www.jnanobiotechnology.com/content/3/1/6
http://en.scientificcommons.org/8443279

[545] Xingmao Jiang, et al. "Aerosol Method for Nano silver-silica Composite Anti-microbial Agent." US Patent US 2009/0175948 A1. Date: Jul. 9, 2009.

[546] Lei Lu, et al. "Silver Nan particles inhibit hepatitis B virus replication." Antiviral Therapy. 2008, vol. 13, pp 253-262.

[547] Xingmao Jiang, et al. "Aerosol Method for Nano silver-silica Composite Anti-microbial Agent." US Patent US 2009/0175948 A1. Date: Jul. 9, 2009.

[548] Vora P. "NANO SILVER INDUCED STEM CELL ACTIVATION."
http://www.space-age.com/StemCellGelPhotoGallery.pdf

[549] Xingmao Jiang, et al. "Aerosol Method for Nano silver-silica Composite Anti-microbial Agent." US Patent US 2009/0175948 A1. Date: Jul. 9, 2009.

[550] Furno F, et al. "Silver nanoparticles and polymeric medical devices: a new approach to prevention of infection?" Journal of Antimicrobial Chemother. 2004, vol. 54(6), pp 1019-1024.

[551] Xingmao Jiang, et al. "Aerosol Method for Nano silver-silica Composite Anti-microbial Agent." US Patent US 2009/0175948 A1. Date: Jul. 9, 2009.

[552] V Edwards-Jones. "The benefits of silver in hygiene, personal care and healthcare." Letters in Applied Microbiology. 2009, vol. 49(2), pp 147-152.

[553] Xingmao Jiang, et al. "Aerosol Method for Nano silver-silica Composite Anti-microbial Agent." US Patent US 2009/0175948 A1. Date: Jul. 9, 2009.

[554] IBID

[555] Jin-Sook Hyun, et al. "Effects of repeated silver nanoparticles exposure on the histological structure and mucins of nasal respiratory mucosa in rats." <u>Toxicology Letters.</u> 2008, vol. 182(1-3), pp 24-228.

[556] Xingmao Jiang, et al. "Aerosol Method for Nano silver-silica Composite Anti-microbial Agent." US Patent US 2009/0175948 A1. Date: Jul. 9, 2009.

[557] IBID

[558] IBID

[559] Nanda M and Saravanan M. "Biosynthesis of silver nanoparticles from *Staphylococcus aureus* and its antimicrobial activity against MRSA and MRSE." <u>Nanomedicine: Nanotechnology, Biology and Medicine.</u> 2009, vol. 5(4), pp 452-456.

[560] Xingmao Jiang, et al. "Aerosol Method for Nano silver-silica Composite Anti-microbial Agent." US Patent US 2009/0175948 A1. Date: Jul. 9, 2009.

[561] Asare N, et al. "Cytotoxic and genotoxic effects of silver Nan particles in testicular cells." <u>Toxicology.</u> 2012, vol. 291(1-3), pp 65-72.

[562] Xingmao Jiang, et al. "Aerosol Method for Nano silver-silica Composite Anti-microbial Agent." US Patent US 2009/0175948 A1. Date: Jul. 9, 2009.

[563] Panacek A, et al. "Silver Colloid Nanoparticles: Synthesis, Characterization, and Their Antibacterial Activity." <u>The Journal of Physical Chemistry</u>. 2006, vol. 110 (33), pp 16248-16253.

[564] Nanda M and Saravanan M. "Biosynthesis of silver nanoparticles from *Staphylococcus aureus* and its antimicrobial activity against MRSA and MRSE." <u>Nanomedicine: Nanotechnology, Biology and Medicine.</u> 2009, vol. 5(4), pp 452-456.

[565] Xingmao Jiang, et al. "Aerosol Method for Nano silver-silica Composite Anti-microbial Agent." US Patent US 2009/0175948 A1. Date: Jul. 9, 2009.

[566] Holladay RJ, Christensen H, and Moeller WD. "Treatment of Humans with Colloidal Silver Composition." US Patent US 7,135,195 B2. Date: Nov 14, 2006.

[567] Marimuthu S, et al. "Evaluation of green synthesized silver nanoparticles against parasites." <u>Parasitol Res.</u> 2011, vol. 108, pp 1541-1549.

[568] Rahman MF, et al. "Expression of genes related to oxidative stress in the mouse brain after exposure to silver-25 Nan particles." <u>Toxicology Letters.</u> 2009, vol. 187(1), pp 15-21.

[569] Galdiero S, et al. "Silver Nanoparticles as Potential Antiviral Agents." <u>Molecules.</u> 2011, vol. 16(10), pp 8894-8918.

[570] Xingmao Jiang, et al. "Aerosol Method for Nano silver-silica Composite Anti-microbial Agent." US Patent US 2009/0175948 A1. Date: Jul. 9, 2009.

[571] Kollef MH, et al. "Silver-Coated Endotracheal Tubes and Incidence of Ventilator-Associated PneumoniaThe NASCENT Randomized Trial." <u>JAMA.</u> 2008, vol. 300(7), pp 805-813.

[572] Vora P. "NANO SILVER INDUCED STEM CELL ACTIVATION." http://www.space-age.com/StemCellGelPhotoGallery.pdf

[573] Yezhelyev MV, et al. "Emerging use of nanoparticals in diagnosis and treatment of breast cancer." <u>The Lancet Oncology.</u> 2006, vol. 7(8), pp 657-667.

[574] Xingmao Jiang, et al. "Aerosol Method for Nano silver-silica Composite Anti-microbial Agent." US Patent US 2009/0175948 A1. Date: Jul. 9, 2009.

[575] IBID

[576] IBID

[577] Xingmao Jiang, et al. "Aerosol Method for Nano silver-silica Composite Anti-microbial Agent." US Patent US 2009/0175948 A1. Date: Jul. 9, 2009.

[578] IBID

[579] Singh M, et al. "Nanotechnology in Medicine and Antibacterial Effect of Silver Nanoparticles." <u>Digest Journal of Nanomaterials and Biostructures.</u> 2008, vol. 3(3), pp 115-122.

[580] Xingmao Jiang, et al. "Aerosol Method for Nano silver-silica Composite Anti-microbial Agent." US Patent US 2009/0175948 A1. Date: Jul. 9, 2009.

[581] IBID

[582] IBID

[583] IBID

[584] Holladay RJ, Christensen H, and Moeller WD. "Treatment of Humans with Colloidal Silver Composition." US Patent US 7,135,195 B2. Date: Nov 14, 2006.

[585] Xingmao Jiang, et al. "Aerosol Method for Nano silver-silica Composite Anti-microbial Agent." US Patent US 2009/0175948 A1. Date: Jul. 9, 2009.

[586] V Edwards-Jones. "The benefits of silver in hygiene, personal care and healthcare." Letters in Applied Microbiology. 2009, vol. 49(2), pp 147-152.

[587] Xingmao Jiang, et al. "Aerosol Method for Nano silver-silica Composite Anti-microbial Agent." US Patent US 2009/0175948 A1. Date: Jul. 9, 2009.

[588] Xingmao Jiang, et al. "Aerosol Method for Nano silver-silica Composite Anti-microbial Agent." US Patent US 2009/0175948 A1. Date: Jul. 9, 2009.

[589] Nanda M and Saravanan M. "Biosynthesis of silver nanoparticles from *Staphylococcus aureus* and its antimicrobial activity against MRSA and MRSE." Nanomedicine: Nanotechnology, Biology and Medicine. 2009, vol. 5(4), pp 452-456.

[590] Xingmao Jiang, et al. "Aerosol Method for Nano silver-silica Composite Anti-microbial Agent." US Patent US 2009/0175948 A1. Date: Jul. 9, 2009.

[591] IBID

[592] Holladay RJ, Christensen H, and Moeller WD. "Treatment of Humans with Colloidal Silver Composition." US Patent US 7,135,195 B2. Date: Nov 14, 2006.

[593] Xingmao Jiang, et al. "Aerosol Method for Nano silver-silica Composite Anti-microbial Agent." US Patent US 2009/0175948 A1. Date: Jul. 9, 2009.

[594] Holladay RJ, Christensen H, and Moeller WD. "Treatment of Humans with Colloidal Silver Composition." US Patent US 7,135,195 B2. Date: Nov 14, 2006.

[595] Xingmao Jiang, et al. "Aerosol Method for Nano silver-silica Composite Anti-microbial Agent." US Patent US 2009/0175948 A1. Date: Jul. 9, 2009.

[596] IBID

[597] IBID

[598] IBID

[599] Vora P. "NANO SILVER INDUCED STEM CELL ACTIVATION." http://www.space-age.com/StemCellGelPhotoGallery.pdf

[600] Holladay RJ, Christensen H, and Moeller WD. "Treatment of Humans with Colloidal Silver Composition." US Patent US 7,135,195 B2. Date: Nov 14, 2006.

[601] Xingmao Jiang, et al. "Aerosol Method for Nano silver-silica Composite Anti-microbial Agent." US Patent US 2009/0175948 A1. Date: Jul. 9, 2009.

[602] IBID

[603] Jun Tian, et al. "Topical Delivery of Silver Nanoparticles Promote Wound Healing." ChemMed Chem. 2007, vol. 2(1), pp 129-136.

[604] Xingmao Jiang, et al. "Aerosol Method for Nano silver-silica Composite Anti-microbial Agent." US Patent US 2009/0175948 A1. Date: Jul. 9, 2009.

[605] Singh M, et al. "Nanotechnology in Medicine and Antibacterial Effect of Silver Nanoparticles." Digest Journal of Nanomaterials and Biostructures. 2008, vol. 3(3), pp 115-122.

[606] IBID

[607] Singh M, et al. "Nanotechnology in Medicine and Antibacterial Effect of Silver Nanoparticles." Digest Journal of Nanomaterials and Biostructures. 2008, vol. 3(3), pp 115-122.

[608] Vora P. "NANO SILVER INDUCED STEM CELL ACTIVATION." http://www.space-age.com/StemCellGelPhotoGallery.pdf

[609] Singh M, et al. "Nanotechnology in Medicine and Antibacterial Effect of Silver Nanoparticles." Digest Journal of Nanomaterials and Biostructures. 2008, vol. 3(3), pp 115-122.

[610] IBID

[611] IBID

[612] Saravanan S, et a.. "Preparation, characterization and antimicrobial activity of a bio-composite scaffold containing chitosan/nano-hydroxyapatite/nano-silver for bone tissue engineering" International Journal of Biological Macromolecules. 2011, vol. 49(2), pp 188-193.

[613] Singh M, et al. "Nanotechnology in Medicine and Antibacterial Effect of Silver Nanoparticles." Digest Journal of Nanomaterials and Biostructures. 2008, vol. 3(3), pp 115-122.

[614] Singh M, et al. "NANOTECHNOLOGY IN MEDICINE AND ANTIBACTERIAL EFFECT OF SILVER NANOPARTICLES." Digest Journal of Nanomaterials and Biostructures. 2008, vol. 3(3), pp 115-122.

[615] Jun Sung Kim, et al. "Antimicrobial effects of silvernanoparticles." Nanomedicine: Nanotechnology, Biology and Medicine. 2007, vol. 3(1), pp 95-101.

[616] Marra V, et al. "Silver Nanoparticles as Potential Antiviral Agents." Molecules. 2011, vol. 16(10), pp 8894-8918.

[617] Morones JR, et al. "The bactericidal effect of silver Nan particles." Nanotechnology. 2005, vol. 16(10), p 2346.

[618] V Edwards-Jones. "The benefits of silver in hygiene, personal care and healthcare." Letters in Applied Microbiology. 2009, vol. 49(2), pp 147-152.

[619] Hee Sun Park, et al. "Attenuation of allergic airway inflammation and hyperresponsiveness in a murine model of asthma by silver nanoparticles." Int J Nanomedicine. 2010, vol. 5, pp 505-515.

[620] Ha Ryong Kim, et al. "Genotoxic effects of silver Nan particles stimulated by oxidative stress in human normal bronchial epithelial (BEAS-2B) cells." Mutation Research/Genetic Toxicology and Environmental Mutagenesis. 2011, vol. 726(2), pp 129-135.

[621] V Edwards-Jones. "The benefits of silver in hygiene, personal care and healthcare." Letters in Applied Microbiology. 2009, vol. 49(2), pp 147-152.

[622] Singh M, et al. "NANOTECHNOLOGY IN MEDICINE AND ANTIBACTERIAL EFFECT OF SILVER NANOPARTICLES." <u>Digest Journal of Nanomaterials and Biostructures.</u> 2008, vol. 3(3), pp 115-122.

[623] Jae Hyuck Sung, et al. "Lung Function Changes in Sprague-Dawley Rats After Prolonged Inhalation Exposure to Silver Nanoparticles." <u>Inhalation Toxicology.</u> 2008, vol. 20(6), pp 567-574.

[624] Singh M, et al. "Nanotechnology in Medicine and Antibacterial Effect of Silver Nanoparticles." <u>Digest Journal of Nanomaterials and Biostructures.</u> 2008, vol. 3(3), pp 115-122.

[625] IBID

[626] IBID

[627] IBID

[628] IBID

[629] "A Blue Man Christmas - Home Grown Silver not Colloidal." http://www.colloidal-silver-information.com/2007/12/

[630] Elechiguerra J, et al. "Interaction of silver nanoparticles with HIV-1." BioMed Central Ltd. 2005

[631] http://jualionicsilver.info/

[632] RM Reynolds. Disorders of sodium balance. BMJ. 2006, vol 332, p 702.

[633] Manunta P, et al. "Physiological Interaction Between α-Adducin and *WNK1-NEDD4L* Pathways on Sodium-Related Blood Pressure Regulation." <u>Hypertension.</u> 2008, vol. 52, pp 366-372.

[634] Bieberdorf FA, Morawski S and Fordtran JS. "Effect of sodium, mannitol, and magnesium on glucose, galactose, 3-O-methylglucose, and fructose absorption in the human ileum." <u>Gastroenterology.</u> 1975, vol. 68(1), pp 58-66.

[635] Stofan JR, et al. "Sweat and Sodium Losses in NCAA Football Players: A Precursor to Heat Cramps?" <u>International Journal of Sport Nutrition and Exercise Metabolism.</u> 2005, vol. 15, pp 64d1-652.

[636] Bieberdorf FA, Morawski S and Fordtran JS. "Effect of sodium, mannitol, and magnesium on glucose, galactose, 3-O-methylglucose, and fructose absorption in the human ileum." <u>Gastroenterology.</u> 1975, vol. 68(1), pp 58-66.

[637] Watanabe S, et al. "Uric Acid, Hominoid Evolution, and the Pathogenesis of Salt-Sensitivity." <u>Hypertension.</u> 2002, vol. 40, pp 355-360.

[638] Rocchini AP, et al. "The effect of weight loss on the sensitivity of blood pressure to sodium in obese adolescents." <u>New England Journal of Medicine.</u> 1989, vol. 321(9), pp 585.

[639] Bruyere O, et al. "Relationship between Bone Mineral Density Changes and Fracture Risk Reduction in Patients Treated with Strontium Ranelate." <u>J of Clin Endocrinology & Metabolism.</u> 2007, vol. 92(8), pp 2076-2081.

[640] Kai Qiu, et al. "Effect of strontium ions on the growth of ROS17/2.8 cells on porous calcium polyphosphate scaffolds." <u>Biomaterials.</u> 2006, vol. 27(8), pp 1277-1286.

[641] Marie PJ, et a. "An Uncoupling Agent Containing Strontium Prevents Bone Loss by Depressing Bone Resorption and Maintaining Bone Formation in Estrogen-Deficient Rats." <u>JBMR</u> 2005, vol. 20(6), pp 1065-1074,

[642] Finlay, et al. "Radioisotopes for the palliation of metastatic bone cancer: a systematic review." <u>The Lancet Oncology.</u> 2005, vol. 6)6_, pp 392-400.

[643] Marie PJ, et al. Mechanisms of Action and Therapeutic Potential of Strontium in Bone. Calcif Tissue Int. 2001, vol. 69, pp 121-129.

[644] Marie PJ, et a. "An Uncoupling Agent Containing Strontium Prevents Bone Loss by Depressing Bone Resorption and Maintaining Bone Formation in Estrogen-Deficient Rats." <u>JBMR</u> 2005, vol. 20(6), pp 1065-1074,

[645] Marie PJ, et a. "An Uncoupling Agent Containing Strontium Prevents Bone Loss by Depressing Bone Resorption and Maintaining Bone Formation in Estrogen-Deficient Rats." <u>JBMR</u> 2005, vol. 20(6), pp 1065-1074,

[646] Marie PJ, et al. "Mechanisms of Action and Therapeutic Potential of Strontium in Bone." <u>Calcif Tissue Int</u>. 2001, vol. 69, pp 121-129.

[647] Wen-Yu Qian, et al. "pH-sensitive strontium carbonate nanoparticles as new anticancer vehicles for controlled etoposide release." <u>Int J Nanomedicine</u>. 2012, vol. 7, pp 5781-5792.

[648] Sila-Asna M, et al. "Osteoblast Differentiation and Bone Formation Gene Expression in Strontium-inducing Bone Marrow Mesenchymal Stem Cell." Kobe J Med Sci. 2007, vol. 53(1), pp 25-35.

[649] Wen-Yu Qian, et al. "pH-sensitive strontium carbonate nanoparticles as new anticancer vehicles for controlled etoposide release." Int J Nanomedicine. 2012, vol. 7, pp 5781-5792.

[650] Marie PJ, et al. "Mechanisms of Action and Therapeutic Potential of Strontium in Bone." Calcif Tissue Int. 2001, vol. 69, pp 121-129.

[651] Meunier, PJ, Roux C. et al. "The Effects of Strontium Ranelate on the Risk of Vertebral Fracture in Women with Postmenopausal Osteoporosis." The New England Journal of Medicine. 2004, vol. 350, pp 459-468.

[652] TH Abdullah, et al. "Garlic Revisited: Therapeutic for the Major Diseases of Our Times?" J Natl Med Assoc. 1988, vol. 80 (4), pp 438-445.

[653] Gabriela Segura, MD.
http://www.sott.net/articles/show/228453-DMSO-The-Real-Miracle-Solution
http://healthnews.benabraham.com/html/dmso_-_the_real_miracle_soluti.html

[654] Rahman K. "Garlic and aging: new insights into an old remedy." Ageing Research Reviews. 2003, vol. 2(1), pp 39-56.

[655] Lin A, et al. "Accumulation of methylsulfonylmethane in the human brain: identification by multinuclear magnetic resonance spectroscopy." Toxicology Letters. 2001, vol. 123(2-3), pp 169-177.

[656] TH Abdullah, et al. "Garlic Revisited: Therapeutic for the Major Diseases of Our Times?" J Natl med Assoc. 1988, vol. 80 (4), pp 438-445.

[657] Gabriela Segura, MD.
http://www.sott.net/articles/show/228453-DMSO-The-Real-Miracle-Solution
http://healthnews.benabraham.com/html/dmso_-_the_real_miracle_soluti.html

[658] Ohki Hiuchi, et al. "Antioxidative Activity of Sulfur-Containing Compounds in *Allium* Species for Human Low-Density Lipoprotein (LDL) Oxidation in Vitro." J Agric Food Chem. 2003, vol. 51 (24), pp 7208-7214.

[659] Martin KA and Barr TL. "Food bar for treating musculoskeletal disorders." US Patent US 2004/0253296 A1. Date: Dec 16, 2004.

[660] Gabriela Segura, MD. http://www.sott.net/articles/show/228453-DMSO-The-Real-Miracle-Solution http://healthnews.benabraham.com/html/dmso_-_the_real_miracle_soluti.html

[661] Castleman, Michael, The Healing Herbs, Rodale Press, 1991, p.179

[662] Rahman K. "Garlic and aging: new insights into an old remedy." Ageing Research Reviews. 2003, vol. 2(1), pp 39-56.

[663] Cheng-Tzu Liu, et al. "Antidiabetic effect of garlic oil but not diallyl disulfide in rats with streptozotocin-induced diabetes." Food and Chemical Toxicology. 2006, vol. 44(8), pp 1377-1384.

[664] Eun Joung Lim, et al. "Methylsulfonylmethane Suppresses Breast Cancer Growth by Down-Regulating STAT3 and STAT5b Pathways." PLoS ONE. 2012. 7(4): e33361. doi:10.1371/journal.pone.0033361.

[665] Gabriela Segura, MD. http://www.sott.net/articles/show/228453-DMSO-The-Real-Miracle-Solution http://healthnews.benabraham.com/html/dmso_-_the_real_miracle_soluti.html

[666] Rahman K. "Garlic and aging: new insights into an old remedy." Ageing Research Reviews. 2003, vol. 2(1), pp 39-56.

[667] Suliman ME, et al. "Plasma sulfur amino acids in relation to cardiovascular disease, nutritional status, and diabetes mellitus in patients with chronic renal failure at start of dialysis therapy." American journal of Kidney diseases. 2002, vol. 40(2), pp 480-488.

[668] Rahman K. "Garlic and aging: new insights into an old remedy." Ageing Research Reviews. 2003, vol. 2(1), pp 39-56.

[669] Rahman K. "Garlic and aging: new insights into an old remedy." Ageing Research Reviews. 2003, vol. 2(1), pp 39-56.

[670] Yu-Yan Yeh and Lijuan Liu. "Cholesterol-Lowering Effect of Garlic Extracts and Organosulfur Compounds: Human and Animal Studies," J Nutr. 2001, vol. 131(3), pp 989S-993S.

[671] Michael J Wargovich. "Diallyl sulfide, a flavor component of garlic (*Allium sativum*), inhibits dimethyihydrazine-induced colon cancer." <u>Carcinogenesis</u>. 1987, vol. 8 (3), pp 487-489.

[672] AT Fleischauer and L Arab. "Garlic and Cancer: A Critical Review of the Epidemiologic Literature." <u>J Nutr.</u> 2001, vol. 131 (3), pp 10325-10405.

[673] BV Howard and D Kritchevsky. "Phytochemicals and Cardiovascular Disease A Statement for Healthcare Professionals From the American Heart Association." <u>Circulation</u>. 1997, vol95, pp 2591-2593.

[674] Castleman, Michael, The Healing Herbs, Rodale Press, 1991, p.179

[675] Cheng-Tzu Liu, et al. "Antidiabetic effect of garlic oil but not diallyl disulfide in rats with streptozotocin-induced diabetes." <u>Food and Chemical Toxicology.</u> 2006, vol. 44(8), pp 1377-1384.

[676] Castleman, Michael, The Healing Herbs, Rodale Press, 1991, p.179

[677] Castleman, Michael, The Healing Herbs, Rodale Press, 1991, p.179

[678] Gabriela Segura, MD.
http://www.sott.net/articles/show/228453-DMSO-The-Real-Miracle-Solution
http://healthnews.benabraham.com/html/dmso_-_the_real_miracle_soluti.html

[679] Hiroyuki Nakagawa, et al. "Growth inhibitory effects of diallyl disulfide on human breast cancer cell lines." <u>Carcinogenesis</u>. 2001, vol. 22 (6), pp 891-897.

[680] Hiroyuki Nakagawa, et al. "Growth inhibitory effects of diallyl disulfide on human breast cancer cell lines." <u>Carcinogenesis</u>. 2001, vol. 22 (6), pp 891-897.

[681] Martin KA and Barr TL. "Food bar for treating musculoskeletal disorders." US Patent US 2004/0253296 A1. Date: Dec 16, 2004.

[682] Martin KA and Barr TL. "Food bar for treating musculoskeletal disorders." US Patent US 2004/0253296 A1. Date: Dec 16, 2004.

[683] Kim LS, et al. "Efficacy of methylsulfonylmethane (MSM) in osteoarthritis pain of the knee: a pilot clinical trial." <u>Osteoarthritis and Cartilage.</u> 2006, vol. 14(3), pp 286-294.

[684] Gabriela Segura, MD.

http://www.sott.net/articles/show/228453-DMSO-The-Real-Miracle-Solution
http://healthnews.benabraham.com/html/dmso_-_the_real_miracle_soluti.html

[685]   Hsing AW, et al. "Allium Vegetables and Risk of Prostate Cancer: A Population-Based Study." JNCI J Natl Cancer Inst. 2002, vol. 94 (21), pp 1648-1651.

[686]   AT Fleischauer and L Arab. "Garlic and Cancer: A Critical Review of the Epidemiologic Literature." J Nutr. 2001, vol. 131 (3), pp 10325-10405.

[687]   Berardesca E, et al. "Combined effects of silymarin and methylsulfonylmethane in the management of rosacea: clinical and instrumental evaluation." Journal of Cosmetic Dermatology. 2008, vol. 7(1), pp 8-14.

[688]   Gabriela Segura, MD.
http://www.sott.net/articles/show/228453-DMSO-The-Real-Miracle-Solution
http://healthnews.benabraham.com/html/dmso_-_the_real_miracle_soluti.html

[689]   IBID

[690]   Rahman K. "Garlic and aging: new insights into an old remedy." Ageing Research Reviews. 2003, vol. 2(1), pp 39-56.

[691]   AT Fleischauer and L Arab. "Garlic and Cancer: A Critical Review of the Epidemiologic Literature." J Nutr. 2001, vol. 131 (3), pp 10325-10405.

[692]   Gabriela Segura, MD.
http://www.sott.net/articles/show/228453-DMSO-The-Real-Miracle-Solution
http://healthnews.benabraham.com/html/dmso_-_the_real_miracle_soluti.html

[693]   McClintock SD, et al. "Attenuation of half sulfur mustard gas-induced acute lung injury in rats." Journal of Applied Toxicology. 2006, vol. 26(2), pp 126-131.

[694]   Rahman K. "Garlic and aging: new insights into an old remedy." Ageing Research Reviews. 2003, vol. 2(1), pp 39-56.

[695]   Castleman, Michael, The Healing Herbs, Rodale Press, 1991, p.179

[696]   Castleman, Michael, The Healing Herbs, Rodale Press, 1991, p.179

[697] Suliman ME, et al. "Plasma sulfur amino acids in relation to cardiovascular disease, nutritional status, and diabetes mellitus in patients with chronic renal failure at start of dialysis therapy." <u>American journal of Kidney diseases.</u> 2002, vol. 40(2), pp 480-488.

[698] Zhang M, et al. "Assessment of methylsulfonylmethane as a permeability enhancer for regional EDTA chelation therapy." <u>Drug Delivery.</u> 2009, vol. 16(5), pp 243-248.

[699] Gabriela Segura, MD.
http://www.sott.net/articles/show/228453-DMSO-The-Real-Miracle-Solution
http://healthnews.benabraham.com/html/dmso_-_the_real_miracle_soluti.html

[700] Gabriela Segura, MD.
http://www.sott.net/articles/show/228453-DMSO-The-Real-Miracle-Solution
http://healthnews.benabraham.com/html/dmso_-_the_real_miracle_soluti.html

[701] Gabriela Segura, MD.
http://www.sott.net/articles/show/228453-DMSO-The-Real-Miracle-Solution
http://healthnews.benabraham.com/html/dmso_-_the_real_miracle_soluti.html

[702] Gabriela Segura, MD.
http://www.sott.net/articles/show/228453-DMSO-The-Real-Miracle-Solution
http://healthnews.benabraham.com/html/dmso_-_the_real_miracle_soluti.html

[703] Diallyl disulfide from Wikipedia, the free encyclopedia.
Amonkar, SV; Banerji, A (1971). "Isolation and characterization of larvicidal principle of garlic". Science 174 (16): 1343–4. doi:10.1126/science.174.4016.1343. PMID 5135721.

[704] Diallyl disulfide. Cayman Chemical.
https://www.caymanchem.com/app/template/Product.vm/catalog/10012582

[705] Cheng-Tzu Liu, et al. "Antidiabetic effect of garlic oil but not diallyl disulfide in rats with streptozotocin-induced diabetes." <u>Food and Chemical Toxicology.</u> 2006, vol. 44(8), pp 1377-1384.

[706] IBID

[707] Corzo-Martinez M, et al. "Biological properties of onions and garlic." <u>Trends in Food Science & Technology.</u> 2007, vol. 18(12), pp 609-625.

[708] IBID

[709] IBID

[710] Rahman K. "Garlic and aging: new insights into an old remedy." <u>Ageing Research Reviews.</u> 2003, vol. 2(1), pp 39-56.

[711] Corzo-Martinez M, et al. "Biological properties of onions and garlic." <u>Trends in Food Science & Technology.</u> 2007, vol. 18(12), pp 609-625.

[712] IBID

[713] IBID

[714] Kun Song and John A. Milner. "The Influence of Heating on the Anticancer Properties of Garlic." <u>J. Nutr</u>. 2001, vol. 131 (3), pp 1054S-1057S

[715] Toyohiko Ariga. "Antithrombotic and anticancer effects of garlic-derived sulfur compounds: A review." <u>BioFactors</u>. 2006, vol. 26 (2), pp 93-103.

[716] Barceloux DG and D Barceloux. "Vanadium." <u>Clinical Toxicology.</u> 1999, vol. 37(2), pp 265-278.

[717] IBID

[718] Ray RS, Rana B, Swami B, Venu V, Chatterjee ., "Vanadium mediated apoptosis and cell cycle arrest in MCF7 cell line." <u>Chemico-Biological Interaction</u>. 2006, vol. 163 (3), pp 239-247

[719] Bhuiyan MS, et al. "Cardioprotective Effect of Vanadyl Sulfate on Ischemia/Reperfusion-Induced Injury in Rat Heart *In vivo* Is Mediated by Activation of Protein Kinase B and Induction of FLICE-Inhibitory Protein." <u>Cardiovascular Drug Reviews.</u> 2008, vol. 26(1), pp 10-23.

[720]   Angelos M Evangelou. "Vanadium in Cancer Treatment." <u>Critical Reviews in Oncology/Hematology.</u> 2002, vol. 42, p. 240-265.

[721]   IBID

[722]   IBID

[723]   Angelos M Evangelou. "Vanadium in Cancer Treatment." <u>Critical Reviews in Oncology/Hematology.</u> 2002, vol. 42, p. 240-265.

[724]   IBID

[725]   IBID

[726]   Bhuiyan MS, et al. "Cardioprotective Effect of Vanadyl Sulfate on Ischemia/Reperfusion-Induced Injury in Rat Heart *In vivo* Is Mediated by Activation of Protein Kinase B and Induction of FLICE-Inhibitory Protein." <u>Cardiovascular Drug Reviews.</u> 2008, vol. 26(1), pp 10-23.

[727]   Klein A, et al. "Sodium Orthovanadate Affects Growth of Some Human Epithelial Cancer Cells (A549, HTB44, DU145)." <u>Folia Biologica.</u> 2008, vol. 56(3-4), pp 115-121(7).

[728]   Angelos M Evangelou. "Vanadium in Cancer Treatment." <u>Critical Reviews in Oncology/Hematology.</u> 2002, vol. 42, p. 240-265.

[729]   Klein A, et al. "Sodium Orthovanadate Affects Growth of Some Human Epithelial Cancer Cells (A549, HTB44, DU145)." <u>Folia Biologica.</u> 2008, vol. 56(3-4), pp 115-121(7).

[730]   Angelos M Evangelou. "Vanadium in Cancer Treatment." <u>Critical Reviews in Oncology/Hematology.</u> 2002, vol. 42, p. 240-265.

[731]   IBID

[732]   Klein A, et al. "Sodium Orthovanadate Affects Growth of Some Human Epithelial Cancer Cells (A549, HTB44, DU145)." <u>Folia Biologica.</u> 2008, vol. 56(3-4), pp 115-121(7).

[733] Hahl H and Kropp W. "Pharmaceutical Compound Consisting of the Magnesium-Vanadium salt of Triglycollamic Acid." Serial No. 4,494. Date Jan. 24, 1925.

[734] Angelos M Evangelou. "Vanadium in Cancer Treatment. <u>Critical Reviews in Oncology/Hematology</u>, 2002, vol. 42, p. 240-265.

[735] IBID

[736] IBID

[737] Pedro I. da S. Maia, et al. "Vanadium complexes with thiosemicarbazones: Synthesis, characterization, crystal structures and anti-*Mycobacterium tuberculosis* activity." <u>Polyhedron.</u> 2009, vol. 28(2), pp 398-406.

[738] Ray RS, Rana B, Swami B, Venu V, Chatterjee M, Vanadium mediated apoptosis and cell cycle arrest in MCF7 cell line, Chemico-Biological Interactions, 2006, vol. 163 (3), pp 239-247.

[739] Angelos M Evangelou. "Vanadium in Cancer Treatment. <u>Critical Reviews in Oncology/Hematology</u>, 2002, vol. 42, p. 240-265.

[740] IBID

[741] IBID

[742] IBID

[743] IBID

[744] IBID

[745] IBID

[746] IBID

[747] Ray RS, Rana B, Swami B, Venu V, Chatterjee M. "Vanadium mediated apoptosis and cell cycle arrest in MCF7 cell line." <u>Chemico-Biological Interactions</u>. 2006, vol. 163 (3), pp 239-247.

[748] Angelos M Evangelou. "Vanadium in Cancer Treatment." <u>Critical Reviews in Oncology/Hematology.</u> 2002, vol. 42, p. 240-265.

[749] Barceloux DG and D Barceloux. "Vanadium." <u>Clinical Toxicology.</u> 1999, vol. 37(2), pp 265-278.

[750] Angelos M Evangelou. "Vanadium in Cancer Treatment." <u>Critical Reviews in Oncology/Hematology.</u> 2002, vol. 42, p. 240-265.

[751] IBID

[752] IBID

[753] Angelos M Evangelou. "Vanadium in Cancer Treatment." <u>Critical Reviews in Oncology/Hematology.</u> 2002, vol. 42, p. 240-265.

[754] IBID

[755] Steven D Ehrlich, NMD. "Vanadium". 6/12/2011. http://www.umm.edu/altmed/articles/vanadium-000330.htm

[756] Angelos M Evangelou. "Vanadium in Cancer Treatment." <u>Critical Reviews in Oncology/Hematology.</u> 2002, vol. 42, p. 240-265.

[757] Drenoo B, et al. "Low doses of zinc gluconate for inflammatory acne." <u>Acta Derm Venereol.</u> 1989, vol. 69(6), pp 541-543.

[758] Prasad AS. "Impact of the Discovery of Human Zinc Deficiency on Health." <u>J Am Coll Nutr.</u> 2009, vol. 28(3), pp 257-265.

[759] IBID

[760] Lambert JC, et al. Prevention of Alterations in Intestinal Permeability Is Involved in Zinc Inhibition of Acute Ethanol-Induced Liver Damage in Mice. JPET. 2003, vol. 305 (3), pp 880-886.

[761] Prasad AS. "Impact of the Discovery of Human Zinc Deficiency on Health." <u>J Am Coll Nutr.</u> 2009, vol. 28(3), pp 257-265.

762 Knoell DL, et al. "Zinc deficiency increases organ damage and mortality in a murine model of polymicrobial sepsis." <u>Crit Care Med.</u> 2009, vol. 37(4), pp 1380-1388.

763 Solomons NW and Russel RM."The interaction of vitamin A and zinc: Implications for human nutrition." <u>American Journal of Clinical Nutrition</u>. 1980, vol. 33 (9), pp 2031-2040.

764 Bush A, et al. "Rapid induction of Alzheimer A beta amyloid formation by zinc." <u>Science</u>. 1994, vol. 265 (5177), pp 1464-1467.

765 Hambidge KM, et al. "Low Levels of Zinc in Hair, Anorexia, Poor Growth, and Hypogeusia in Children." <u>Pediatric Research</u>. 1972, vol. 6, pp 868-874.

766 Prasad AS. "Impact of the Discovery of Human Zinc Deficiency on Health." <u>J Am Coll Nutr.</u> 2009, vol. 28(3), pp 257-265.

767 Prasad AS. "Impact of the Discovery of Human Zinc Deficiency on Health." <u>J Am Coll Nutr.</u> 2009, vol. 28(3), pp 257-265.

768 Sandstead HH, et al. History of Zinc as Related to Brain Function. J Nutr. 2000, vol. 130 (2), pp 496S-502S.

769 IBID

770 Humphries L, et al. "Zinc deficiency and Eating disorders." <u>Journal of Clinical Psychiatry.</u> 1989, vol. 50(12), pp 456-459.

771 Coogan TP, et al. "Cadmium-induced DNA strand damage in cultured liver cells: Reduction in cadmium genotoxicity following zinc pretreatment." <u>Toxicology and Applied Pharmacology</u>. 1992, vol. 113 (2), pp 227-233.

772 Maggini, et al. "Essential Role of Vitamin C and Zinc in Child Immunity and Health." <u>J of International Medical Research.</u> 2010, vol. 38(2), pp 386-414.

773 CF Walker and RE Black. "ZINC AND THE RISK FOR INFECTIOUS DISEASE." <u>Annual Review of Nutrition</u>. 2004, vol. 24, pp 255-275.

774 Aggarwal R, et al. "Role of Zinc Administration in Prevention of Childhood Diarrhea and Respiratory Illnesses: A Meta-analysis." <u>Pediatrics</u>. 2007, vol. 119 (6), pp 1120-1130.

[775] Prasad AS. "Impact of the Discovery of Human Zinc Deficiency on Health." J Am Coll Nutr. 2009, vol. 28(3), pp 257-265.

[776] Solomons NW and Russel RM. "The interaction of vitamin A and zinc: Implications for human nutrition." American Journal of Clinical Nutrition. 1980, vol. 33 (9), pp 2031-2040.

[777] Prasad AS. "Impact of the Discovery of Human Zinc Deficiency on Health." J Am Coll Nutr. 2009, vol. 28(3), pp 257-265.

[778] LM Klevay. "Coronary heart disease: the zinc/copper hypothesis." Am J Clin Nutr. 1975, vol. 28 (7), pp 764-774.

[779] Berger MM. "Zinc: A Key Pharmaconutrient in Critically Ill Patients?" JPEN 2008, vol. 32(5), pp 582-584.

[780] Addy M, Richards J and Williams G. "Effects of a zinc citrate mouthwash on dental plaque and salivary bacteria." J of Clinical Periodontology. 1980, vol. 7(4), pp 309-315.

[781] Aggarwal R, et al. "Role of Zinc Administration in Prevention of Childhood Diarrhea and Respiratory Illnesses: A Meta-analysis." Pediatrics. 2007, vol. 119 (6), pp 1120-1130.

[782] Humphries L, et al. "Zinc deficiency and Eating disorders." Journal of Clinical Psychiatry. 1989, vol. 50(12), pp 456-459.

[783] Prasad AS. "Impact of the Discovery of Human Zinc Deficiency on Health." J Am Coll Nutr. 2009, vol. 28(3), pp 257-265.

[784] Solomons NW and Russel RM. "The interaction of vitamin A and zinc: Implications for human nutrition." American Journal of Clinical Nutrition. 1980, vol. 33 (9), pp 2031-2040.

[785] Nasser, et al. Antiviral activity of influenza virus M1 zinc finger peptides. Journal Virol. 1996. Vp; 70 (12), pp 8639-8644.

[786] Prasad AS. "Impact of the Discovery of Human Zinc Deficiency on Health." J Am Coll Nutr. 2009, vol. 28(3), pp 257-265.

[787] Prasad AS. "Impact of the Discovery of Human Zinc Deficiency on Health." J Am Coll Nutr. 2009, vol. 28(3), pp 257-265.

[788]   Solomons NW and Russel RM. "The interaction of vitamin A and zinc: Implications for human nutrition." <u>American Journal of Clinical Nutrition</u>. 1980, vol. 33 (9), pp 2031-2040.

[789]   Prasad AS. "Impact of the Discovery of Human Zinc Deficiency on Health." <u>J Am Coll Nutr.</u> 2009, vol. 28(3), pp 257-265.

[790]   Solomons NW and Russel RM. "The interaction of vitamin A and zinc: Implications for human nutrition." <u>American Journal of Clinical Nutrition</u>. 1980, vol. 33 (9), pp 2031-2040.

[791]   IBID

[792]   IBID

[793]   Prasad AS. "Impact of the Discovery of Human Zinc Deficiency on Health." <u>J Am Coll Nutr.</u> 2009, vol. 28(3), pp 257-265.

[794]   IBID

[795]   IBID

[796]   IBID

[797]   IBID

[798]   IBID

[799]   Banudevi, et al. "Protective effect of zinc on *N*-methyl-*N*-nitrosourea and testosterone-induced prostatic intraepithelial neoplasia in the dorsolateral prostate of Sprague Dawley rats." <u>Exp Biol Med.</u> 2011, vol. 236(9), pp 1012-1021.

[800]   Lothar Rink and Klaus-Helge. "Zinc-altered Immune Function." Institute of Immunology, University Hospital, Technical University of Aachen, Aachen, Germany.
11th International Symposium on Trace Elements in Man and Animals   Abstracts jn.nutrition.org at NIH Lib Acquisitions Unit/MSC 1150 on August 20, 2008 http://ods.od.nih.gov/attachments/Abstracts.pdf#search="gaba gamma-aminobutyric acid"

[801]   Beauman JG. "Genital herpes: a review." <u>Am Fam Physician</u>. 2005, vol. 72 (8), pp 1527-1524.

[802] Prasad AS. "Impact of the Discovery of Human Zinc Deficiency on Health." J Am Coll Nutr. 2009, vol. 28(3), pp 257-265.

[803] Maggini, et al. "Essential Role of Vitamin C and Zinc in Child Immunity and Health." J of International Medical Research. 2010, vol. 38(2), pp 386-414.

[804] Prasad AS. "Impact of the Discovery of Human Zinc Deficiency on Health." J Am Coll Nutr. 2009, vol. 28(3), pp 257-265.

[805] Knoell DL, et al. "Zinc deficiency increases organ damage and mortality in a murine model of polymicrobial sepsis." Crit Care Med. 2009, vol. 37(4), pp 1380-1388.

[806] Fraker PJ, et al. "Regeneration of T-cell helper function in zinc-deficient adult mice." PNAS 1979, vol. 75(11).

[807] Prasad AS and Kucuk O. "Zinc in Cancer Prevention." Cancer and Metastasis Reviews. 2002, vol. 21(3-4), pp 291-295.

[808] Leitzmann MF, et al. "Zinc Supplement Use and Risk of Prostate Cancer." JNCI 2003, vol. 95(13), pp 1004-1007.

[809] Giovannucci EL. Zinc Supplement Use and Risk of Prostate Cancer. JNCI J Natl Cancer Inst. 2003, vol. 95 (13), pp 1004-1007.

[810] Scozzafava A, et al. Anticancer and antiviral sulfonamides. Current medicinal Chemistry. 2003, vol. 10 (11), pp 925-953.

[811] Dr. Chase's Recipes Information for Everybody, 1902, Stanton and Van Vliet Co., Chicago, p. 137.

[812] Spice Williams–Crosby. "Sick Soil, Sick Plants, Sick People." Doctoral Dissertation submitted to University of Natural Medicine. http://www.spice-of-life.com/columns/dissertation/UNM_PhD_Dissertation_and_Updated_References.pdf

[813] Berger MM. "Zinc: A Key Pharmaconutrient in Critically Ill Patients?" JPEN 2008, vol. 32(5), pp 582-584.

[814] F. Batmaghelidj, The Wonders of Water: Amazing Secrets of Health and Wellness. F Batmaghelidj - Tren.net
http://scholar.google.com/scholar?hl=en&q=water+dehydration+angina&btnG=&as_sdt=1%2C6&as_sdtp=

[815] The information on salt intake is taken from Dr. Batmanghelidj's book, "Water: Rx for a Healthier Pain-Free Life".

[816] F. Batmanghelidj, MD. "Neurotransmitter Histamine: an Alternative View Point. Foundation for the Simple in Medicine." Sci. Med. Simplified. 1990, vol 1, pp 8-39.
http://www.watercure.com/pdf/neurotranmitter_histamine.pdf

[817] R Susanna Jr., et al. "The relation between intraocular pressure peak in the water drinking test and visual field progression in glaucoma." Br J Ophthalmol. 2005, vol 89, pp 1298-1301.

[818] Wynckel A, et al. "Intestinal calcium absorption from mineral water."Mineral and Electrolyte Metabolism. 1997, vol 23 (2), pp 88-92.

[819] Meunier PJ, et al. "Consumption of a high calcium mineral water lowers biochemical indices of bone remodeling in postmenopausal women with low calcium intake." Osteoporosis International. 2005, vol 16, issue 10, pp 1203-1209.

[820] Schoppen S, et al. "A Socium-Rich Carbonated Mineral Water Reduces Cardiovascular Risk in Postmenopausal Women." J. Nutr. 2004, vol 134, no 5, pp 1058-1063.

[821] Marie-France Muller. Colloidal Minerals And Trace Elements: How To Restore The Body's Natural Vitality. Healing Arts Press. Inner Traditions International. Rochester, VT. Copyrighted 2002. English translation, 2005. Page 1.
http://books.google.com/books?hl=en&lr=&id=bP7BaltR9a8C&oi=fnd&pg=PR7&dq=illite+french+green+clay+therapeutic+fulvic+acid&ots=t33JaAm22w&sig=4abE5t_EzgPNMdFU9gqHh5bLdAo#v=onepage&q&f=false

[822] Dekker J and Medlen CE. "Fulvic acid and its use in the Treatment of Various Conditions." US Patent US 6,569,900 B1 Date: May 27, 2003.

[823] IBID

[824] IBID

825 Yamada P, et al. "Inhibitory Effect of Fulvic Acid Extracted from Canadian Sphagnum Peat on Chemical Mediator Release by RBL-2H3 and KU812 Cells." Bioscience, Biotechnology, and Biochemistry. 2007, vol. 71(5), pp 1294-1305.

826 Carrasco-Gallardo C, et al. Shilajit: A Natural Phytocomplex with Potential Procognitive Activity. International Journal of Alzheimer's Disease. 2012, article ID 674142, 4 pagesdoi:10.1155/2012/674142.

827 Dekker J and Medlen CE. "Fulvic acid and its use in the Treatment of Various Conditions." US Patent US 6,569,900 B1 Date: May 27, 2003.

828 Trckova M, et al. "Peat as a feed supplement for animals: a review." Vet Med-Czech. 2005(8), pp 361-377.

829 Chong-Hua Chen, et al. "The effect of humic acid on the adhesibility of neutrophils." Thrombosis Research. 2002, vol. 108(1), pp 67-76.

830 Pant K, et al. Shilajit: A Humic Matter Panacea for Cancer. International Journal of Toxicological and Pharmacological Research. 2012, vol. 4 (2), pp 17-25. http://www.ijtpr.com/PDF%20all%20edtions%20IJTPR/Vol4/Issue2/IJTPR,Vol4,Issue2,Article2.pdf

831 About Humic - Fulvic Substances II. Advanced Bioceuticals. 2005, pp 1-38. http://www.curezone.org/upload/Blogs/Your_Enchanted_Gardener/Humic_Fulvic_Substances_II.pdf#page=8

832 Pongprapansiri T, Chatikavanit P, and Boonchuen S. "Novel Composition for the Treatment of Wounds and Skin Care." US Patent US 2010/0284951 A1. Date: Nov 11, 2010.

833 Pongprapansiri T, Chatikavanit P, and Boonchuen S. "Novel Composition for the Treatment of Wounds and Skin Care." US Patent US 2010/0284951 A1. Date: Nov 11, 2010.

834 Pongprapansiri T, Chatikavanit P, and Boonchuen S. "Novel Composition for the Treatment of Wounds and Skin Care." US Patent US 2010/0284951 A1. Date: Nov 11, 2010.

835 Trivedi NA, et al. Research Paper - Effect of shilajit on blood glucose and lipid profile in alloxaninduced diabetic rats. Indian Journal of Pharmacology. 2004, vol. 36 (6). https://tspace.library.utoronto.ca/handle/1807/3954

[836] Pongprapansiri T, Chatikavanit P, and Boonchuen S. "Novel Composition for the Treatment of Wounds and Skin Care." US Patent US 2010/0284951 A1. Date: Nov 11, 2010.

[837] Cho-Rok Jung, et al. Osteoblastic differentiation of mesenchymal stem cells by mumie extract. Drug Development Research. 2002, vol. 57 (3), pp 122-133.

[838] Pant K, et al. "Shilajit: A Humic Matter Panacea for Cancer." International Journal of Toxicological and Pharmacological Research. 2012, vol. 4 (2), pp 17-25.

[839] About Humic - Fulvic Substances II. Advanced Bioceuticals. 2005, pp 1-38. http://www.curezone.org/upload/Blogs/Your_Enchanted_Gardener/Humic_Fulvic_Substances_II.pdf#page=8

[840] Sherry L, et al. "Carbohydrate Derived Fulvic Acid: An *in vitro* Investigation of a Novel Membrane Active Antiseptic Agent Against *Candida albicans* Biofilms." Front Microbiol. 2012, vol. 3, p 116.

[841] Pant K, et al. "Shilajit: A Humic Matter Panacea for Cancer." International Journal of Toxicological and Pharmacological Research. 2012, vol. 4 (2), pp 17-25.

[842] Carrasco-Gallardo C, et al. "Shilajit: A Natural Phytocomplex with Potential Procognitive Activity." International Journal of Alzheimer's Disease. 2012, article ID 674142, 4 pagesdoi:10.1155/2012/674142.

[843] Pongprapansiri T, Chatikavanit P, and Boonchuen S. "Novel Composition for the Treatment of Wounds and Skin Care." US Patent US 2010/0284951 A1. Date: Nov 11, 2010.

[844] Trivedi NA, et al. "Research Paper - Effect of shilajit on blood glucose and lipid profile in alloxaninduced diabetic rats." Indian Journal of Pharmacology. 2004, vol. 36 (6).

[845] Pongprapansiri T, Chatikavanit P, and Boonchuen S. "Novel Composition for the Treatment of Wounds and Skin Care." US Patent US 2010/0284951 A1. Date: Nov 11, 2010.

[846] Dekker J and Medlen CE. "Fulvic acid and its use in the Treatment of Various Conditions." US Patent US 6,569,900 B1 Date: May 27, 2003.

[847] Petralia R. "Nutraceutical Beverage.", US Patent US 2012/0214756 A. Date: 8/23/2012

848 Yinzhang Cui. "Cellular regeneration attributed to Fulvic acid electrolyte."
Advanced Bioceuticals. Humic Acid, 1 (1991).
http://www.thewaterlady.com/uploads/Cellular_regeneration_attributed_to_Ful
vic_acid_electrolyte.pdf
http://info-archive.com/fulvic_resp.htm

849 About Humic - Fulvic Substanced II. Advanced Bioceuticals. 2005.
Yuan, Shenyuan; Fulvic Acid, 4 1988; in Application of Fulvic acid and its
derivatives in the fields of agriculture and medicine; First Edition: June 1993
http://www.curezone.org/upload/Blogs/Your_Enchanted_Gardener/Humic_Fulvi
c_Substances_II.pdf#page=8

850 Guofan, Tang. "Cellular regeneration attributed to Fulvic acid electrolyte."
Advanced Bioceuticals. Jianngxi, 3 (1984).
http://www.thewaterlady.com/uploads/Cellular_regeneration_attributed_to_Ful
vic_acid_electrolyte.pdf

851 http://info-archive.com/fulvic_resp.htm

852 Dekker J and Medlen CE. "Fulvic acid and its use in the Treatment of Various
Conditions." US Patent US 6,569,900 B1 Date: May 27, 2003.

853 Yuan, Shenyuan. Fulvic Acid Minerals Information. "It's all about oxygen and
fulvic trace elements."Fulvic Acid, 4 1988; in Application of Fulvic acid and its
derivatives in the fields of agriculture and medicine ; First Edition: June 1993
http://www.vitalo2.com/fulvic%20medicinal%20oxygen%20fulvic%20trace%20el
ements%20colloidal%20minerals%20magnesium%20nutrients%20supplements%
201206.htm

854 http://info-archive.com/fulvic_resp.htm

855 Pant K, et al. "Shilajit: A Humic Matter Panacea for Cancer." International
Journal of Toxicological and Pharmacological Research. 2012, vol. 4 (2), pp 17-25.

856 Gadd Gmand Griffiths AJ. "Microorganisms and Heavy Metal Toxicity."
Microbial Ecology. 1978, vol. 4, pp 303-317.

857 Fulvic Acid Minerals Information. It's all about oxygen and fulvic trace
elements.

http://www.vitalo2.com/fulvic%20medicinal%20oxygen%20fulvic%20trace%20el
ements%20colloidal%20minerals%20magnesium%20nutrients%20supplements%
201206.htm

[858] Pant K, et al. "Shilajit: A Humic Matter Panacea for Cancer." <u>International Journal of Toxicological and Pharmacological Research</u>. 2012, vol. 4 (2), pp 17-25.

[859] Pongprapansiri T, Chatikavanit P, and Boonchuen S. "Novel Composition for the Treatment of Wounds and Skin Care." US Patent US 2010/0284951 A1. Date: Nov 11, 2010.
http://www.google.com/patents?hl=tl&lr=&vid=USPATAPP12436796&id=g9bbAA
AAEBAJ&oi=fnd&dq=fulvic+humic+acid+athlete%27s+foot+gangrene&printsec=a
bstract#v=onepage&q=fulvic%20humic%20acid%20athlete's%20foot%20gangren
e&f=false

[860] Pant K, et al. "Shilajit: A Humic Matter Panacea for Cancer." <u>International Journal of Toxicological and Pharmacological Research</u>. 2012, vol. 4 (2), pp 17-25.

[861] Dekker J and Medlen CE. "Fulvic acid and its use in the Treatment of Various Conditions." US Patent US 6,569,900 B1 Date: May 27, 2003.

[862] Dekker J and Medlen CE. "Fulvic acid and its use in the Treatment of Various Conditions." US Patent US 6,569,900 B1 Date: May 27, 2003.

[863] Agarwal SP, et al. "Complexation of Furosemide with Fulvic Acid Extracted from Shilajit: A Novel Approach." <u>Drug Development and Industrial Pharmacy.</u> 2008, vol. 34(5), pp 506-611.

[864] Rung-Jiun Gau, et al. "Humic Acid Suppresses the LPS-Induced Expression of Cell-Surface Adhesion Proteins through the Inhibition of NF-κB Activation." <u>Toxicology and Applied Pharmacology</u>. 2000, vol. 166 (1), pp 59-67.

[865] Bingwen Su. "Cellular regeneration attributed to Fulvic acid electrolyte." <u>Advanced Bioceuticals</u>. Jiangxi Humic Acid, 3 (1985).
http://www.thewaterlady.com/uploads/Cellular_regeneration_attributed_to_Ful
vic_acid_electrolyte.pdf

[866] Ganapathy R. "In Vitro Analysis of the Anti-influenza Virus Activity of Pomegranate Products and Fulvic Acid." Master's Thesis. University of Tennessee, 2009.

[867] Pant K, et al. "Shilajit: A Humic Matter Panacea for Cancer." <u>International Journal of Toxicological and Pharmacological Research</u>. 2012, vol. 4 (2), pp 17-25.

[868]   Zraly Z, et al. "Effect of Humic Acids on Lead Accumulation in Chicken Organs and Muscles." <u>Acta Vet Brno.</u> 2008, vol. 77, pp 439-445.

[869]   Kaushik DI, Gupta V, Bansal P, Khokra SI. "Therapeutic Potentials of Shilajit Rasayan". <u>International Journal of Pharmaceutical and Clinical Research</u>. 2009, vol. 1 (2), pp47-49

[870]   http://info-archive.com/fulvic_resp.htm

[871]   About Humic - Fulvic Substances II. <u>Advanced Bioceuticals</u>. 2005, pp 1-38. http://www.curezone.org/upload/Blogs/Your_Enchanted_Gardener/Humic_Fulvic_Substances_II.pdf#page=8

[872]   Petralia R. "Nutraceutical Beverage.", US Patent US 2012/0214756 A. Date: 8/23/2012

[873]   Reported claims of effective treatment of Symptoms. Info Archive Site http://www.info-archive.com/Fulv%20claims.htm

[874]   Petralia R. "Nutraceutical Beverage.", US Patent US 2012/0214756 A. Date: 8/23/2012

[875]   ibid

[876]   Cho-Rok Jung, et al. "Osteoblastic differentiation of mesenchymal stem cells by mumie extract." <u>Drug Development Research</u>. 2002, vol. 57 (3), pp 122-133.

[877]   Ganapathy R. "In Vitro Analysis of the Anti-influenza Virus Activity of Pomegranate Products and Fulvic Acid." Master's Thesis. University of Tennessee, 2009.

[878]   http://info-archive.com/fulvic_resp.htm

[879]   Ganapathy R. "In Vitro Analysis of the Anti-influenza Virus Activity of Pomegranate Products and Fulvic Acid." Master's Thesis. University of Tennessee, 2009.

[880]   Petralia R. "Nutraceutical Beverage.", US Patent US 2012/0214756 A. Date: 8/23/2012

881 Pongprapansiri T, Chatikavanit P, and Boonchuen S. "Novel Composition for the Treatment of Wounds and Skin Care." US Patent US 2010/0284951 A1. Date: Nov 11, 2010.

882 Chong-Hua Chen, et al. "The effect of humic acid on the adhesibility of neutrophils." Thrombosis Research. 2002, vol. 108(1), pp 67-76.

883 He, Shenyi, et al. About Humic - Fulvic Substances II. "Humic acid in Jiangxi Province." Advanced Bioceuticals. 2005, pp 1-38, 1 (1982) http://www.curezone.org/upload/Blogs/Your_Enchanted_Gardener/Humic_Fulvic_Substances_II.pdf#page=8

884 Petralia R. "Nutraceutical Beverage.", US Patent US 2012/0214756 A. Date: 8/23/2012

885 Yuan, Shenyuan. "Fulvic Acid Minerals Information. It's all about oxygen and fulvic trace elements."
Fulvic Acid, 4 1988; in Application of Fulvic acid and its derivatives in the fields of agriculture and medicine ; First Edition: June 1993.

886 Yuan, Shenyuan. "Fulvic Acid Minerals Information. It's all about oxygen and fulvic trace elements."
Fulvic Acid, 4 1988; in Application of Fulvic acid and its derivatives in the fields of agriculture and medicine ; First Edition: June 1993.

887 Chong-Hua Chen, et al. "The effect of humic acid on the adhesibility of neutrophils." Thrombosis Research. 2002, vol. 108(1), pp 67-76.

888 Dekker J and Medlen CE. "Fulvic acid and its use in the Treatment of Various Conditions." US Patent US 6,569,900 B1 Date: May 27, 2003.

889 Sabi R, et al. "Carbohydrate-derived Fulvic acid (CHD-FA) inhibits Carrageenan-induced inflammation and enhances wound healing: efficacy and Toxicity study in rats." Drug Development Research. 2012, vol. 73(1), pp 18-23.

890 http://info-archive.com/fulvic_resp.htm

891 Fulvic and enzymes – Pardue, H.L, Townshend, A., Clere, J.T., VanderLinden (Eds.), (1990, May 1). Analytica chimica Acta, Special Issue, Humic and Fulvic compounds, 232 (1), 1-235. (Amsterdam, Netherlands: Elsevier Science Publishers) 24 Increase assimilation- Buffle http://www.enerex.ca/articles/fulvic_acid_the_miracle_molecule.pdf

[892]   Pant K, et al. "Shilajit: A Humic Matter Panacea for Cancer." <u>International Journal of Toxicological and Pharmacological Research</u>. 2012, vol. 4 (2), pp 17-25.

[893]   IBID

[894]

http://www.curezone.org/upload/Blogs/Your_Enchanted_Gardener/Humic_Fulvic_Substances_II.pdf#page=8

[895]   Dr. Richard A. Drucker. "The Gift of Naturally Prolonged Healthy and Sustained Life, Organic, Homeostatic, Soil-Based Fulvic Acid and the Intraceliuiar Energy System." <u>The American Chiropractor.</u> 2008

[896]   Schlickewei, Dr. W., (1993). "Influence of humate on calcium hydroxyapatite implants." <u>Arch Orthop Trauma Surg.</u> 112:275-279,

[897]   Radha Ganapathy. "In Vitro Analysis of the Anti-influenza Virus Activity of Pomegranate Products and Fulvic Acid." Master's Thesis, University of Tennessee, 2009.

[898]   Schlickewei, Dr. W., (1993). "Influence of humate on calcium hydroxyapatite implants." <u>Arch Orthop Trauma Surg.</u> 112:275-279,

[899]   Schlickewei, Dr. W., (1993). "Influence of humate on calcium hydroxyapatite implants." <u>Arch Orthop Trauma Surg.</u> 112:275-279,

[900]   IBID

[901]   Vucskits AV, et al. "Effect of fulvic and humic acids on performance, immune response and thyroid function in rats." <u>Journal of Animal Physiology and Animal Nutrition.</u> 2010, vol. 94(6), pp 721-728.

[902]   Dekker J and Medlen CE. "Fulvic acid and its use in the Treatment of Various Conditions." US Patent US 6,569,900 B1 Date: May 27, 2003.

[903]   Rung-Jiun Gau, et al. "Humic Acid Suppresses the LPS-Induced Expression of Cell-Surface Adhesion Proteins through the Inhibition of NF-κB Activation." <u>Toxicology and Applied Pharmacology</u>. 2000, vol. 166 (1), pp 59-67.

[904]   http://info-archive.com/fulvic_resp.htm

[905] Dekker J and Medlen CE. "Fulvic acid and its use in the Treatment of Various Conditions." US Patent US 6,569,900 B1 Date: May 27, 2003.

[906] Pant K, et al. Shilajit: A Humic Matter Panacea for Cancer. International Journal of Toxicological and Pharmacological Research. 2012, vol. 4 (2), pp 17-25.

[907] http://info-archive.com/fulvic_resp.htm

[908] Pant K, et al. Shilajit: A Humic Matter Panacea for Cancer. International Journal of Toxicological and Pharmacological Research. 2012, vol. 4 (2), pp 17-25.

[909] He, Shenyi, et al. "Outpatient medical hospital studies on thyroid tumors, some cancerous, showed that injections with a special humic extract was 90% successful in stopping tumor growth and diminishing size of tumors, with 80% of patients having complete cures." Humic acid in Jiangxi Province, 1 (1982) http://www.curezone.org/upload/Blogs/Your_Enchanted_Gardener/Humic_Fulvi c_Substances_II.pdf#page=8

[910] http://info-archive.com/fulvic_resp.htm

[911] Pant K, et al. Shilajit: A Humic Matter Panacea for Cancer. International Journal of Toxicological and Pharmacological Research. 2012, vol. 4 (2), pp 17-25.

[912] Fulvic Acid Minerals Information. It's all about oxygen and fulvic trace elements. http://www.vitalo2.com/fulvic%20medicinal%20oxygen%20fulvic%20trace%20el ements%20colloidal%20minerals%20magnesium%20nutrients%20supplements% 201206.htm

[913] Pant K, et al. Shilajit: A Humic Matter Panacea for Cancer. International Journal of Toxicological and Pharmacological Research. 2012, vol. 4 (2), pp 17-25.

[914] IBID.

[915] IBID

[916] Dangers of chlorine in relation to humic substances. Info Archive Site. http://www.info-archive.com/fulvwarning.htm

[917] Fulvic Acid The Miracle Molecule. Morningstar Minerals http://www.enerex.ca/articles/fulvic_acid_the_miracle_molecule.pdf

[918] Fulvic Acid Minerals Information. Info Archive Site.

http://info-archive.com/fulvic_nutrition.htm

[919] Yinzhang Cui, Humic Acid, 1 (1991)
http://office.enerex.ca/articles/fulvic_humic_acid.pdf#page=5

[920] Yuan, Shenyuan. "Fulvic acid and Humic extract topical use and bath therapies show amazing clinical results." Fulvic Acid Minerals Information. Fulvic acid 4 1988; in Application of Fulvic acid and its derivatives in the fields of agriculture and medicine; First Edition: June 1993.

[921] IBID

[922] Jingrong Chen et al. "Fulvic acid and Humic extract topical use and bath therapies show amazing clinical results." Fulvic Acid Minerals Information. Jiangxi. 1984, vol. 2.

[923] Wilson, et al. "Review on shilajit used in traditional Indian medicine." Journal of Ethnopharmacology. 2011, vol. 136(1), pp 1-9.

[924] Carrasco-Gallardo C, et al. Shilajit: A Natural Phytocomplex with Potential Procognitive Activity. International Journal of Alzheimer's Disease. 2012, article ID 674142, 4 pagesdoi:10.1155/2012/674142.

[925] Mohan L, et al. "Evaluation of the Anxiolytic Activity of NR-ANX-C (a Polyherbal Formulation) in Ethanol Withdrawal-Induced Anxiety Behavior in Rats." Evidence-Based Complementary and Alternative Medicine. 2011, vol. 2011, Article ID 327160, 7 pages.

[926] Mohd Aamir Mirza, et al. "Shilajit: An Ancient Panacea." International Journal of Current Pharmaceutical Review and Research. 2010, vol. 1 (1), pp 2-11.

[927] Meena H, et al. "*Shilajit:* A panacea for high-altitude problems." Int J Ayurveda. 2010, vol. 1 (1), pp 27-40.

[928] Surapaneni DK, et al. "Shilajit attenuates behavioral symptoms of chronic fatigue syndrome by modulating the hypothalamic–pituitary–adrenal axis and mitochondrial bioenergetics in rats." Journal of Ethnopharmacology. 2012, vol. 143(1), pp 91-99.

[929] Meena H, et al. "*Shilajit:* A panacea for high-altitude problems." Int J Ayurveda. 2010, vol. 1 (1), pp 27-40.

[930] Carrasco-Gallardo C, et al. "Shilajit: A Natural Phytocomplex with Potential Procognitive Activity." <u>International Journal of Alzheimer's Disease</u>. 2012, article ID 674142, 4 pagesdoi:10.1155/2012/674142.

[931] Meena H, et al. "*Shilajit:* A panacea for high-altitude problems." <u>Int J Ayurveda</u>. 2010, vol. 1 (1), pp 27-40.

[932] IBID

[933] Mohd Aamir Mirza, et al. "Shilajit: An Ancient Panacea." <u>International Journal of Current Pharmaceutical Review and Research</u>. 2010, vol. 1 (1), pp 2-11.

[934] IBID

[935] Meena H, et al. "*Shilajit:* A panacea for high-altitude problems." <u>Int J Ayurveda</u>. 2010, vol. 1 (1), pp 27-40.

[936] IBID

[937] Agarwal SP, et al. "Complexation of Furosemide with Fulvic Acid Extracted from Shilajit: A Novel Approach." <u>Drug Development and Industrial Pharmacy</u>. 2008, vol. 34(5), pp 506-611.

[938] Meena H, et al. "*Shilajit:* A panacea for high-altitude problems." <u>Int J Ayurveda</u>. 2010, vol. 1 (1), pp 27-40.

[939] IBID

[940] IBID

[941] IBID

[942] Mohd Aamir Mirza, et al. "Shilajit: An Ancient Panacea." <u>International Journal of Current Pharmaceutical Review and Research</u>. 2010, vol. 1 (1), pp 2-11.

[943] IBID

[944] IBID

[945] IBID

[946] Meena H, et al. "*Shilajit:* A panacea for high-altitude problems." <u>Int J Ayurveda</u>. 2010, vol. 1 (1), pp 27-40.

[947]   IBID

[948]   Mohd Aamir Mirza, et al. "Shilajit: An Ancient Panacea." <u>International Journal of Current Pharmaceutical Review and Research</u>. 2010, vol. 1 (1), pp 2-11.

[949]   IBID

[950]   Meena H, et al. *Shilajit:* A panacea for high-altitude problems." <u>Int J Ayurveda</u>. 2010, vol. 1 (1), pp 27-40.

[951]   IBID

[952]   Mohd Aamir Mirza, et al. "Shilajit: An Ancient Panacea." <u>International Journal of Current Pharmaceutical Review and Research</u>. 2010, vol. 1 (1), pp 2-11.

[953]   Hua Yin, et al. "Glycine- and GABA-mimetic Actions of Shilajit on the Substantia Gelatinosa Neurons of the Trigeminal Subnucleus Caudalis in Mice." <u>Korean J Physiol Pharmacol</u>. 2011, vol. 15 (5), pp 285-289.

[954]   Julius Goepp, MD. "Reverse Mitochondrial Damage Potent Molecular Energizers for Lifelong Health." <u>Life Extension magazine</u>. 2010.

[955]   Meena H, et al. *Shilajit:* A panacea for high-altitude problems." <u>Int J Ayurveda</u>. 2010, vol. 1 (1), pp 27-40.

[956]   IBID

[957]   IBID

[958]   Mohd Aamir Mirza, et al. "Shilajit: An Ancient Panacea." <u>International Journal of Current Pharmaceutical Review and Research</u>. 2010, vol. 1 (1), pp 2-11.

[959]   Pant K, et al. "Shilajit: A Humic Matter Panacea for Cancer." <u>International Journal of Toxicological and Pharmacological Research</u>. 2012, vol. 4 (2), pp 17-25.

[960]   Meena H, et al. *Shilajit:* A panacea for high-altitude problems." <u>Int J Ayurveda</u>. 2010, vol. 1 (1), pp 27-40.

[961]   Pant K, et al. "Shilajit: A Humic Matter Panacea for Cancer." <u>International Journal of Toxicological and Pharmacological Research</u>. 2012, vol. 4 (2), pp 17-25.

[962]   Mohd Aamir Mirza, et al. "Shilajit: An Ancient Panacea." <u>International Journal of Current Pharmaceutical Review and Research</u>. 2010, vol. 1 (1), pp 2-11.

[963]   Pant K, et al. Shilajit: A Humic Matter Panacea for Cancer. International Journal of Toxicological and Pharmacological Research. 2012, vol. 4 (2), pp 17-25.

[964]   Mohd Aamir Mirza, et al. "Shilajit: An Ancient Panacea." <u>International Journal of Current Pharmaceutical Review and Research</u>. 2010, vol. 1 (1), pp 2-11.

[965]   Pant K, et al. "Shilajit: A Humic Matter Panacea for Cancer." <u>International Journal of Toxicological and Pharmacological Research</u>. 2012, vol. 4 (2), pp 17-25.

[966]   IBID

[967]   Meena H, et al. "*Shilajit:* A panacea for high-altitude problems." <u>Int J Ayurveda</u>. 2010, vol. 1 (1), pp 27-40.

[968]   Mohd Aamir Mirza, et al. "Shilajit: An Ancient Panacea." <u>International Journal of Current Pharmaceutical Review and Research</u>. 2010, vol. 1 (1), pp 2-11.

[969]   Permien T and Lagaly G. "THE RHEOLOGICAL AND COLLOIDAL PROPERTIES OF BENTONITE DISPERSIONS IN THE PRESENCE OF ORGANIC COMPOUNDS V. BENTONITE AND SODIUM MONTMORILLONITE AND SURFACTANTS." <u>Clays and Clay Minerals.</u> 1995, vol. 43(2), pp 229-236.

[970]   Permien T and Lagaly G. "THE RHEOLOGICAL AND COLLOIDAL PROPERTIES OF BENTONITE DISPERSIONS IN THE PRESENCE OF ORGANIC COMPOUNDS V. BENTONITE AND SODIUM MONTMORILLONITE AND SURFACTANTS." <u>Clays and Clay Minerals.</u> 1995, vol. 43(2), pp 229-236.

[971]   Pronovost AD. "Compositions and methods for treating lacerations, abrasions, avulsions, burns, ulcers, and cases of excessive bleeding." US Patent no. US 2009/0148502 A. Date: Jun 11, 2009.

[972]   Phillips TD. "Dietary clay in the chemoprevention of aflatoxin-induced disease." <u>Toxicol Sci.</u> 1999, vol. 52(1), pp 118-126.

[973]   Chan C, et al. "Evaluation of the antiviral activity of different modifications of nano-bentonite clay against the Human Influenza (H3N2) Virus, Avian Influenza (H5N1) Virus, and the Human Immunodeficiency Virus." AMCOL International. London

[974] Pronovost AD. "Compositions and methods for treating lacerations, abrasions, avulsions, burns, ulcers, and cases of excessive bleeding." US Patent no. US 2009/0148502 A. Date: Jun 11, 2009.

[975] Pronovost AD. "Compositions and methods for treating lacerations, abrasions, avulsions, burns, ulcers, and cases of excessive bleeding." US Patent no. US 2009/0148502 A. Date: Jun 11, 2009.

[976] Ding Yue-hai. Effect of Montmorillonite Powder in Treatment of 40 Cases of Infant Diarrhea. Journal of Yangtze University Natural Science Edition. 2011-09.

[977] Tewodros K, et al. "Defluoridation of drinking water by using calcium loaded bentonite." Ethiop J Health Sci. 2006, vol. 16(2), pp 101-108.

[978] Pronovost AD. "Compositions and methods for treating lacerations, abrasions, avulsions, burns, ulcers, and cases of excessive bleeding." US Patent no. US 2009/0148502 A. Date: Jun 11, 2009.

[979] Gomes C and Silva J. "Minerals and clay minerals in medical geology." Applied Clay Science. 2007, vol. 36(1-3), pp 4-21.

[980] Charlotte Chan, et al. "Evaluation of the antiviral activity of different modifications of nano-bentonite clay against the Human Influenza (H3N2) Virus, Avian Influenza (H5N1)." Amcol International. London, UK.

[981] Ijagbemi CO, et al. "Montmorillonite surface properties and sorption characteristics for heavy metal removal from aqueous solutions." Journal of hazardous Material. 2009, vol. 166 (1), pp 538-546.

[982] Chan C, et al. "Evaluation of the antiviral activity of different modifications of nano-bentonite clay against the Human Influenza (H3N2) Virus, Avian Influenza (H5N1) Virus, and the Human Immunodeficiency Virus." AMCOL International. London

[983] Odom IE. "Method of applying magnesium-rich calcium montmorillonite to skin for oil and organic compound sorption." US Patent 5,840,320. Date Nov 24, 1998.

[984] Lawrence J. "Preparation for Regulating Lower Bowel Function." European Patent Specification Application nu: 00907330.5. International Publication nu: WO 00/050056 (31.082000 Gazette 2000/35). Date: 23.02.2000.

[985] Pronovost AD. "Compositions and methods for treating lacerations, abrasions, avulsions, burns, ulcers, and cases of excessive bleeding." US Patent no. US 2009/0148502 A. Date: Jun 11, 2009.

[986] Zhang H, et al. "Sorption characteristics of Pb(II) on alkaline Ca-bentonite." Applied Clay Science. 2012, vol. 65-66, pp 21-23.

[987] Szanto Z and Papp L. "Effect of the different factors on the iontophoretic delivery of calcium ions from bentonite." Journal of Controlled Release. 1998, vol. 56(1-3), pp 239-247.

[988] Zhang Chao-Xian and Qin Yong-mei. "Effects of montmorillonite powder on epidermal growth factor contents in stomach of rats with acetic gastric ulcer." West China Journal of Pharmaceutical Sciences. 2008-06.

[989] Khan SA. "Sorption of the long-lived radionuclides cesium-134, strontium-85 and cobalt-60 on bentonite." Journal of Radioanalytical and Nuclear Chemistry. 2003, vol. 258(1), pp 3-6.

[990] Carretero MI, et al. "Chapter 11.5 Clays and Human Health." Developments in Clay Science. 2006, vol. 1, pp 717-741.

[991] Pronovost AD. "Compositions and methods for treating lacerations, abrasions, avulsions, burns, ulcers, and cases of excessive bleeding." US Patent no. US 2009/0148502 A. Date: Jun 11, 2009.

[992] SH Emami-Razavi, et al. "EFFECT OF BENTONITE ON SKIN WOUND HEALING: EXPERIMENTAL STUDY IN THE RAT MODEL." Acta Medica Iranica. 2006, vol. 44 (4), pp 235-240.

[993] BKG Theng. "Interactions between montmorillonite and fulvic acid." Geoderma. 1976, vol. 15 (3), pp 243-251.

LT Evans and EW Russel. "THE ADSORPTION OF HUMIC AND FULVIC ACIDS BY CLAYS." Journal of Soil Science. 1959, vol. 10 (1), pp 119-132.

[994] Yuancai Dong and Si-Shen Feng. "Poly(d,l-lactide-co-glycolide)/montmorillonite nanoparticles for oral delivery of anticancer drugs." Biomaterial. 2005, vol. 26 (30), pp 6068-6076.

[995] Carretero MI, et al. "Chapter 11.5 Clays and Human Health." <u>Developments in Clay Science.</u> 2006, vol. 1, pp 717-741.

[996] Chan C, et al. "Evaluation of the antiviral activity of different modifications of nano-bentonite clay against the Human Influenza (H3N2) Virus, Avian Influenza (H5N1) Virus, and the Human Immunodeficiency Virus." AMCOL International. London.

[997] http://www.herbalremedies.com/reswhatmakpa.html

[998] Hu XR, et al. "Study on the mechanism of the interaction between montmorillonite and bacterium." <u>Xao Xue Xue Bao</u>. 2002, vol. 37 (9), pp 718-720.

[999] Charlotte Chan, et al. "Evaluation of the antiviral activity of different modifications of nano-bentonite clay against the Human Influenza (H3N2) Virus, Avian Influenza (H5N1)." Amcol International. London, UK.

[1000] http://www.naturalnews.com/022422.html

[1001] Williams LB, et al. "CHEMICAL AND MINERALOGICAL CHARACTERISTICS OF FRENCH GREEN CLAYS USED FOR HEALING." <u>Clays and Clay Minerals</u>. 2008, vol. 56 (4), pp 437-452.

[1002] Williams LB and Haydel SE. "Evaluation of the medicinal use of clay minerals as antibacterial agents." <u>International Geology Review</u>. 2010, vol. 52 (7-8), pp 745-770.

[1003] http://www.naturalnews.com/022422.html

[1004] Haydel SE, et al. "Broad-spectrum in vitro antibacterial activities of clay minerals against antibaiotic-susceptible and antibiotic-resistant bacterial pathogens." <u>J Antimicrob Chemother.</u> 2008, vol. 61 (2) ,pp 353-36.1

[1005] FG Israfilova, "Experience in the multi-modal therapy of acne, including volcano mud applications and cosmetic procedures," <u>Vestn Dermatol Venerol.</u> 1989, vol. 2 pp 56–7.

[1006] EM Ivanov, OV Shakirova, NS Zhuravskaia, "Ultraviolet irradiation of blood and peloid therapy of patients with chronic bronchitis," <u>Vopr Kurortol Fizigter Lech Fiz Kult.</u> 2001, vol. 4, pp 13–7.

[1007] E Proksch et al. "Bathing in a magnesium-rich Dead Sea salt solution improves skin barrier function, enhances skin hydration, and reduces inflammation in atopic dry skin," Int J Dermatol. 2005, vol. 44, pp 151–7.

[1008] C Comacchi, J Hercogova, "A single mud treatment induces normalization of stratum corneum hydration, transepidermal water loss, skin surface pH, and sebum content in patients with seborrhoeic dermatitis," Journal of European Academic Dermatology. 2004, vol. 18, pp 372–4.

[1009] AM Beer et al. "The effect of peat components on endocrine and immunological parameters and on trace elements," Department of Natural Cure, Blankenstein Hospital, Hattingen, Germany, Clin Lab. 2001, vol. 47, pp 161–7.

[1010] S Bellometti, L Galzigna, "Function of the hypothalamic adrenal axis in patients with fibromyalgia syndrome undergoing mud-pack treatment," Int J Clin Pharmacol Res. 1999, vol. 19, pp 27–33.

[1011] EB Vvgodner, SN Serebriakov, AS Bobkova, "Non-medicinal methods of correction of immune disorders in peptic ulcer patients," Ter Arkh. 1991, vol. 63, pp 78–81.

[1012] O Kristof et al. "Analgesic efficacy of the serial application of a sulfurated mud bath at home," Forsch Komplementarmed Klass Naturheilkd. 2000, vol. 7, pp 233–6.

[1013] M Delfino et al. "Experimental study on the efficacy of thermal muds of Ischia Island combined with balneotherapy in the treatment of psoriasis vulgaris with plaques," Clin Ter. 2003, vol. 154, pp 167–71.

[1014] AK Strelis, NA Zhivotiagina, MA Kuz'michev, "Changes in the bronchial tree under the influence of pelotherapy in patients with pulmonary tuberculosis," Probl Tuberk. 1989, vol. 9, pp 16–8.

[1015] S Sukenik et al. "Mud pack therapy in rheumatoid arthritis." Clin Rheumatol. 2000, vol. 11, pp 243–7.

[1016] C Ekmekcioglu et al. "Effect of Sulfur Baths on Antioxidative Defense Systems, Peroxide Concentrations and Lipid Levels in Patients with Degenerative Osteoarthritis," Complementary and Classical Natural Medicine. 2002, vol. 9, pp 216–220.

[1017] M Mesrogli et al. "Successful prevention of adhesions using peat and humic acids," <u>Zentralbl Gynakol</u> 1991, vol. 113, pp 583–90.